'Why Us, Lord?'

'Why Us, Lord?'

'The trauma of infertility: personal experiences'

Joy Cooke

Pickering Paperbacks

For the privacy of the couples and families who shared their stories, fictitious names have been substituted in all instances except where the author writes of her own experience.

First Published
by Pickering & Inglis,
3 Beggarwood Lane,
Basingstoke, Hants RG23 7LP,
United Kingdom

British Library Cataloguing in Publication

Cooke, Joy
Why us Lord?: the trauma of infertility: a personal experience.
1. Infertility—Religious aspects—Christianity
I. Title
261.5′6 BT732

ISBN 0-7208-0636-4

Typeset by Brian Robinson, North Marston, Bucks
Printed and bound in Great Britain by Hazell Watson and Viney Limited, Aylesbury, Bucks.

Contents

This book is dedicated to
our very dear friends Dave and Jenny,
who had to wait so long for their son, Jonathan.

Acknowledgements

I am indebted to so many people for the help they have given me in writing this book. Firstly I would thank my husband Ian, who bullied me into doing it; he is my severest critic and is invariably right, and he has been a tremendous support to me throughout. My thanks go also to Jane Davies, who painstakingly deciphered my work for typing and had infinite patience when I repeatedly changed the script. To my father and uncle, both of whom kept me on my toes for accuracy, and to the latter for finding out and treating the cause of our infertility.

Finally, my greatest debt is to all those who so readily shared their stories, re-living painful experiences, honestly examining and exposing their thoughts and feelings for me and for you. My very real thanks go to these people, for without them I would never have written the book.

Foreword

The pain of childlessness is different from any other kind of pain. It has different stages, and phases. Yet, those who are childless and those who are wanting to help, find little available to help them understand this unique and specially hurtful situation.

As Joy Cooke says, in sharing her own experiences: 'We shunned the help we were offered, because none had trodden our road. Those who came to comfort had children of their own. How could they understand the depth of our feelings?'

For Joy and her husband, their dilemma was enhanced by the fact that they were practising Christians, and could not accept all that was suggested or taught by well meaning people who operated from a point of view very different from their own.

The obvious first question they had to face as Christians was, 'Why was God denying us this simple request (for a child)? We were not asking for anything abnormal or extravagant. A loving God, who is himself a father, would surely not withold this precious gift ... I blamed God ... then I felt guilty for this unprecedented feeling ...'

In her book Joy does not hesitate to open up some of these difficult questions she and her husband faced, and to share with the reader the way in which God helped them through so that at last they were willing to live without children if this was what God had planned for them—but reaching this place came only after long and bitter struggle, disappointments, and growing to understand themselves as a married couple in a far deeper way than they had before.

In seeking to come to terms with her own childlessness, Joy is also forced to consider modern baby-making techniques, ranging from artificial insemination by husband right through to test-tube babies and surrogate motherhood, and she seeks to come to a Christian decision on how they relate to her as someone wanting to live biblically. Her Christian thinking on the matters that currently are being discussed in the Warnock report are timely and helpful.

This is a book to help you understand—it is a book to read if you do not have children, and it is a book to read if you do. It will equip you to talk to any in your church who face the pain of childlessness but do not know a Christian with whom they can share their pain and where they could find comfort. Reading this book will equip you to understand, care and love practically and biblically.

Anne Townsend

Anne Townsend was editor of Family magazine and is now Director of CARE Trust.

Introduction

'Could you tell me, please, where I might find a book on infertility?' The assistant stared blankly at me and then said, 'What is infertility?' I blanched visibly, swallowed hard and wondered where to begin. In the end I simply said, 'It is the inability to have children.' She continued to look blank so I said, 'Maybe there is someone else who would know?' As I spoke an older assistant detached herself from the crowd around the desk and came over.

'I think you've come to the wrong place. What you want is a medical bookshop, where you will get a book that will explain all the facts about infertility.' She smiled sympathetically. It was my turn to look blank. 'But I don't need a book on the facts, *I know* the facts. What I want is a Christian book that tells me how Christians deal with the subject.'

'Oh, we have nothing like that here.' I looked around the massive shop and then turned back to stare at the assistant. I couldn't resist saying, 'Maybe Christians don't have that sort of problem?' 'Oh yes,' she replied, 'I'm sure they do, but nobody would write a book on such a subject.' I made a quick exit from the shop.

Unfortunately this experience is not an isolated one. Enter most Christian book shops and ask for a book on sex or death and you will be directed immediately to the relevant section, without so much as a blush or furtive glance. Here you will find a large selection of books written as textbooks for the learned, guidance for Mr Average, or a biography or autobiography dealing with personal angles of the issue. Not so with the subject of infertility. At best, you will be pointed to the section on family and marriage, where you may find an isolated paragraph here and there. And if, like us, the subject is near to your heart and you are already suffering from its indignities, you will doubtless abandon the search and either opt for support from secular books and societies, or you will simply abandon the search altogether and retire into your own secluded nest to be alone.

Hopefully Christians will soon be able to deal as openly with this subject of infertility as we are now able to talk about earlier taboo subjects such as sex and death. Indeed, the present trend is towards frankness and many Christian magazines have carried recent articles or personal stories.

When I began to write this book, three years ago, there was a wall of silence and embarrassment surrounding infertility. In books on marriage we found the question of starting a family was discussed, but seldom was the question of childlessness ever mentioned. In the few books where it was introduced, it received but a brief mention, often recommending adoption as the Christian alternative. But what of the disappointments and heartaches of waiting, the long medical round, the endless hoping? My husband and I used to joke that there is no such thing as 'family planning', only family prevention.

We have been through the bitter experience of finding ourselves unable to have children easily and it is this, along with the experiences of other couples, some of whom are success stories, others not, which I have recorded in this book. I did not intend to enter the moral religious debate on the subject, (indeed what book can be exhaustive on a topical subject such as this, which is making new strides almost on a weekly basis?) This is a collection of personal stories. But medical, moral and ethical matters appear throughout because they affect our lives, choices and decisions and for that reason cannot be excluded.

I hope it will encourage those who are finding it difficult to have the baby they want. You will identify yourself many times over in these accounts and I hope that you will derive strength and comfort from them. I also hope to enlighten other Christians, who might not have seriously considered the implications of infertility and might not wish to wade through a text-book on the subject, so that they can be more understanding and supportive.

Joy Cooke
1984

1. Marriage: Beginning Life Together

In The Beginning

Take my hand, in yours,
My love,
As I give myself to you.

Knit one, Purl one,
The stitches should be two
But knit two together
And then it's back to one.

One body
One mind
One person

Marriage
A perfect union

Our love will last and stand the course
Our love will weather the storms
Our love will blossom and grow to maturity
Our love will stand in time.

We do not know
What we will face
What will be the better,
the worse,
the richer,
the poorer,

the sickness,
the health,
but together we'll take them on.

Take my hand in yours,
My love,
As I give myself to you.

'How many children would you like?' asked Ian as he put down his fork.

'Sixteen.' I said.

'Fine,' replied Ian, intent once more on his moussaka. The happy laughter and chatter of people enjoying an evening out in a Greek family restaurant swirled around us, as our eyes met momentarily across the small table. Ian smiled slowly before continuing. 'It sounds very Biblical and I suppose you want them all to have Biblical names?'

'Naturally,' I promptly responded. 'And the last shall be called Hezekiah.' My eyes laughed at my sorely tried fiancé as he replied, 'But, of course.'

So it became a standing joke between us that we should have sixteen children and that the last should be called Hezekiah. Our families joined in the laughter of those early days of our engagement; it wasn't until much later that we were to discover that having one child was going to be difficult enough.

I come from a large family, at least by today's standards. There were four children, neatly arranged in a girl-boy-girl-boy sequence, spanning about six years. To me, my home was a happy place and family life an enjoyable experience, so I grew up with the desire to become a wife and mother.

From my middle school years, I had my eyes fixed on this, however, I wanted to do well and to please my parents so I applied myself religiously to my studies. I aimed high and despite the long training and the hard work involved I applied to study medicine at University.

Needless to say this meant commitment to long hours of study which left little room for a whirlwind social life. Yet I did manage to be involved in our Church youth group and to have a couple of boyfriends! It was not until I was twenty, that I began to think seriously about my original deep-rooted desire.

By this time I had changed careers. Science never was very intelligible to me and physics finally short-circuited me, so that I lost my offer of a place to study medicine. I was very disappointed, although not really all that surprised as my physics teacher had warned me of impending disaster. Already, I had thought of alternatives, so it was not too difficult to switch to a career in dietetics.

Just before I started at London University on a four year course, a new face appeared at our church. A young man had moved to our area and was looking for a place to worship. His sister recommended him to attend our church, but he decided to visit a church further down the road. Within minutes of leaving home, he joined a queue of traffic, which was being delayed by major roadworks and so as the hour of eleven chimed he hastily parked the car and slipped into our church after all. He stayed.

A year later we were sitting in that Greek restaurant planning a family.

Ian soon whittled away our prospective family tree and beat me down to a modest four. However, lower than that I would not go and in no way would I accept the norm of 2.3!

'A boy for me, a girl for you!' he teased. 'That's all we need. It's practical, economical, it's even logical.' 'You're biased!' I retorted, for he came from a small family, having only one older sister. He definitely wanted a family, but not a whole clan.

During those early days of our engagement, amidst the rush of wedding plans, we, like so many others, were busy discovering each other's minds. We talked about anything and everything as it occurred, testing each thought, questioning each answer, probing and prodding as we sought to learn about the other. Never had we talked as much as we did then.

Into many of these discussions and debates the idea of a family would present itself and affect our views. When we discussed alcohol, it led to wondering whether we would feel differently when we had children; the question of budgeting led to discussions on pocket money and so on. It was so natural.

When we told my parents that we would like to get married, they put no obstacles in our way. As we talked together about our plans my father did make one stipulation, I should finish my training. As it happened we were all in one mind about this, because I had only just started my four year course in dietetics and we all felt that I should have some sort of career, even though I was to be married. I knew that I would probably need to work from the financial viewpoint, both before and after having a family. Ian had just moved from a job in landscape management to a lecturing post and this was not well paid.

But there was no doubt in my mind that my place was in the home. During the long student vacations, and later when I gave up work for a trial period, we found that our lifestyles were much more settled and enjoyable. However, financial burdens were big, so, I agreed fairly happily to complete my course, and also to do a year of dietetic experience. Four and a half years of voluntary childlessness stretched before me.

Ian was not too worried about the wait. Like most men he was involved in so many other things, his new job, his new wife, his new youth group and so on.

So, after six fast-talking fast-planning months, in which we learnt to agree on many things, although not on the extent of our family tree, we were married in our Baptist Church. It was a real family wedding as my father was minister, so he played two roles; the giving away and the joining together. And it was there, before a large congregation of family, friends and neighbours, that we heard again the familiar words of the marriage ceremony and took them to ourselves making our vows for life.

> 'Marriage is a holy estate instituted by God and commended in Scripture as honourable to all who enter it lawfully and in true affection . . .
>
> It was ordained for the increase of mankind, and

> that children might be brought up in the fear and nurture of the Lord.
>
> It was ordained for the companionship, help and comfort which husband and wife ought to have of each other.
>
> It was ordained for the welfare of human society, which can be strong and happy only where the marriage bond is held in honour.

In turn we each gave our vow, solemnly committing ourselves to each other.

The words that we had heard and said were to come back to us many years later, when in despair over our infertility we had to examine them again and question the whole purpose of marriage. In the future we would look very closely at the 'causes for which it was ordained' and we would weigh up the ethics of some of the medical aspects against the vows that we had made.

But that was for the future. We were married and delighted with each other. Marriage was better, and worse, than expected so we spent the first year ironing out the wrinkles and knocking each other into a much pleasanter shape.

It was great fun as we learnt to discard our individual identities and make one person. We led very full lives at work and at church and what spare time we had was spent decorating an enormous flat we had rented over the college where Ian worked. Happy we certainly were and if occasionally I wished we didn't have to wait so long for a family it was a transient thought, usually arising from the news that a friend was pregnant.

As my graduation approached we began to shed the carefree student image and I was decidedly getting impatient to reach my goal.

A step towards this comfortable state was to take out a mortgage and buy a house. We tramped from property to property, but we found our dream to be somewhat elusive. We were just beginning to think that we would be better off without the burden of respectability, when we found it:

an end-of-terrace Victorian house, which was up for auction. We had two weeks in which to get it surveyed and to get a mortgage agreement in our hand!

We moved in; I graduated and we entered the last phase of our four year plan.

However impatient I was to set up my nursery I knew that we had another year for renovations to bring order out of chaos. My working year would provide the wherewithal as well as the experience which everyone said would stand me in good stead for the future.

As it happened, I spent two years at a small private hospital and a further year in a large teaching hospital, so I certainly got my experience! For the first six months I applied myself to my career, but before long my mind began to wander. At times when work was slack, I would find myself idly looking at the nearest calendar and doing complicated mental arithmetic. Endless futile calculations to see when I could become pregnant, when I could leave work, when I could have a baby.

As Ian knocked down walls, plastered holes, built cupboards and painted ceilings, he listened to my latest calculation and muttered incoherent replies. Finally the message reached him. 'We'd better get started love, if you're ever going to have Hezekiah. I wouldn't like the poor little chap to get left behind just because you're too old.' He side-stepped a painty hug and laughed at my excitement, but deep down I knew that he too was excited. It had been a good four years with just the two of us, but now we were more than ready for children.

2. Miscarriage: The Experience of Losing a Baby

The Miscarriage

It's all over now
I feel deflated
Like a balloon
Punctured prematurely.
Lifeless
Pointless

I know that every cloud has a silver lining
that at least I can get pregnant
that I will be a better person
that trials lead to maturity
that testing means you love me Lord.

I know that early miscarriages are commonplace
that every other woman has had one
that I am lucky to have been pregnant
that next time I will fall quicker
that the foetus must have been malformed.

I know all this and much more
I can answer with truth and hope
And yet

Why do I feel so low
want to weep uncontrollably
to raise my fists to heaven?

Right now

Deep inside

Is a void so big.

That was our baby, Lord
Conceived from our love
With your divine help and blessing

That was a human life
We have marvelled at its conception
its growth
the wonder of its creation.
We have hugged our happy secret
We have loved our unborn babe.

Gone
Finished

What would it have been like?
He or she?
Dark or fair?
Good natured? How futile. IT is GONE

And we are empty

This is a passing sadness
A temporary thing
But very real, Lord, very real

Do you understand, Lord?
You who faced so much?
Does anyone really understand?
They say they do.
They all offer advice, encouragement
Did they ever feel this barrenness?

I think you did, Lord
I am beginning to understand how you felt
Alone, with no-one to share your lonely vigil

No-one to really understand
Your separation
You suffered much more
But the same sentiments

I understand
You understand

So it is to your arms I come, Lord
Hold me tight
Weep my tears, your tears
Share my sorrow, your sorrow

And then, in the morning
Lift me high
That I might fly
Like an eagle
Soaring
Giving Glory
To the Father
Angry fists
Prised open
Raised hands
Giving praise

As you did

Re-furbish my spirit
Give me hope
Mend me
Make me
Lord of my sorrow.

What excitement and joy we experienced in those first few months, as in the satisfaction of our God-given natural desires, we knew we were also fulfilling one of God's purposes for our lives. It was a time full of hope and we found our love deepening. It was to stand us in good stead for the months ahead, and I later came to thank God for it.

The months came and went and my menstrual cycle

continued its repetitive course. As each period started I would find myself noting the date in my diary, then counting seven days and nine months. More hopeful calculations done in that first moment of disappointment and then forgotten for the rest of the month. It really didn't worry me too much at first, because I knew that many people had to wait a while.

By the sixth month, however, I was very impatient. In my naiveté it had never occurred to me that it could take 'so long'. After all, it only needed one egg and one sperm, it couldn't be that difficult. I certainly wasn't thinking about fertile periods, hormones and so on.

A talk with my mother clarified a few salient points. I went out and bought a thermometer. We became a little more scientific as I took my temperature every morning, before I got out of bed and recorded it on a scrap of paper. I should really have recorded the daily temperature on a chart, as the aim of the exercise is to pinpoint the moment when ovulation occurs. I learnt that in a typical textbook case, the normal body temperature (BBT*) drops approximately 0.4 degrees centigrade before ovulation takes place and then rises by 0.5 degrees after ovulation. This is the fertile time of the month, when an egg is released from the ovary and travels up the fallopian tube towards the uterus. I discovered that it is during the journey from the ovary to the uterus that the egg must be fertilized by the male sperm. So as soon as the temperature changes took place I would alert Ian that it was all systems go. It never occurred to us that we shouldn't then make love every night for a week. What a lot we had to learn!

As time went by, I began to experience what so many women talk about, the 'black week'. After each menstrual period, the cycle would begin again and I would look forward to a new month, a fresh chance with my optimism at its highest. As the time of ovulation approached, I would become excited, expectant, hopeful. In some strange way the day my temperature rose would be a day of elation, I would feel as though I was walking on air and I would be convinced that this month everything would be different.

Until the tedium of regulated, pre-determined intercourse began to wear on us, I even enjoyed the thought that 'this is the day' and the fun of 'trying again'. Then, just before a period, I would begin to get tense. I would start to count the days, wondering if and when the dreaded period would start. Mentally, I ticked off each clear day and longed for the end of the month with a kind of desperate optimism, holding back from the possible disappointment of another failure.

As the signs of pre-menstrual tension set in, I would hope fervently that I was mistaken and try to find excuses for why I was feeling low, weepy, headachy, bloated and so on. Then one day I would know that it was all over for this month, another failure, another wasted opportunity. For the first few days of each period, black depression would settle on me and I would be really unbearable to live with.

Ian, who would also be disappointed, got sick of the whole thing, knowing that the relief which came when I emerged into a fresh cycle, was likely to be as short-lived as the last.

After eight months of trying, twenty-eight, twenty-nine, thirty, thirty-one days passed. I never went over my regular twenty eight day cycle: there was only one answer, I must be pregnant! By the end of that week I was getting nausea during the day. This confused me because I thought it was supposed to be *morning* sickness! However, I didn't argue, at last I was pregnant.

We hugged our five-week old secret to ourselves and rejoiced in this new life, our flesh and blood. We talked about breaking the exciting news to our families and went and bought a knitting pattern for a baby's matinee jacket to send to Ian's mother and a 'Grandma's Boasting Book' to give to mine. We were like a couple of kids with a huge secret, bursting to tell everyone we met, yet wanting to keep it all to ourselves.

Ian's eyes would sparkle as he met mine across the supper table and he would hug me very tightly when I went out to work and tell me to look after his child. My step was light and I even remember skipping to the Underground station at eight o'clock in the morning. A secret smile played about my lips.

My joy lasted another week and then one day at work, I began to miscarry. Utterly dismayed but unsure of what I should do, I decided to wait until the evening and then go to surgery. Ian picked me up from the station and drove me down and then left me to go in, while he waited in the car. How I wish he had come in with me.

My own much-respected doctor was on holiday, so I was seen by a young locum. I explained the situation and asked him what I should do. I was not prepared for his answer.

'Run around the block.' He said quite starkly, before going on to explain, 'An early abortion like this is quite common and is nature's way of discharging a malformed foetus, so it's best to get rid of it as quickly as possible.' His eyes shifted uncomfortably as he read the disbelief in mine.

'But can't you stop it? I thought it was possible to do something positive. I mean . . .' My voice petered out and I sat speechless before him, a lump in my throat and tears threatening to fall.

'I'm sorry. There's a lot of conflicting advice about what to do, but most doctors agree that at such an early stage it is better to let nature do her work.' Suddenly, I saw a man in a dilemma. As he began to ask me routine questions like my age, how long we had been married, how long we had been trying and so on, I realized that he was stalling for time. He was embarrassed by my distress, pessimistic about the outcome of this pregnancy, anxious to get through his busy surgery and unsure about how to soften the blow. I put him out of his misery by leaving the surgery and taking my tears to my waiting husband.

We wanted that baby. We had longed for this time and already I was thinking of the new life within me, of the foetus that was half an inch long and whose heart was already formed and beating. I ignored the doctor's advice and spent a quiet evening with my feet up, hoping that he was wrong. He wasn't.

By nine o'clock that evening I was having severe cramp pains and felt very sick. An hour later, I didn't know where to put myself, the painkillers hadn't worked and my optimism was waning fast. Ian phoned the doctor, and the senior partner happened to be on duty. 'He says you are to take painkillers every four hours, to have a hot bath and then take a hot water bottle to bed and sleep it off. We are to ring the surgery first thing in the morning and tell him how you are. He also said that if you can't sleep I should give you a sleeping tablet, but we haven't got any.'

By the next morning the cramp had stopped and I didn't know what was happening. Ian phoned the surgery, and was put through to another locum. He was encouraging and told me to potter around the house saying he would call later in the day. It was mid-afternoon when the door-bell rang, and Ian showed the doctor into the living-room. He smiled politely at me and then asked to see the patient. I explained that I was the patient. He looked startled.

'But I was told that you are miscarrying. Why aren't you in bed?'

'Because you told me to potter around quietly until you came.' I was annoyed at his attitude.

'It wasn't me you spoke to. I am from an agency that sends locum doctors to do house calls when a practice is short-staffed.' He sat down next to me as he spoke and smiled kindly. 'Tell me,' he said, 'do you want this baby?' He reeled a bit under the force of my reply and then said 'You should be on complete bed-rest.'

By then it was too late to save the pregnancy but nevertheless I went to bed to let my body recover. Five different doctors, with five different opinions: no wonder we were confused and left wondering whether, in fact the pregnancy could have been saved. I was bitterly disappointed and so was Ian and we found that all the comforting words of friends and relatives did little to console us.

We tried to pray, even though we weren't as close to the Lord as we should have been, but we just ended up weeping and berating the Lord for allowing this mishap. A Christian friend visiting us at the time told us that we should rejoice in all things and that we should thank God for allowing us to suffer. After she had gone I tried, but it wasn't from the heart and so we were left feeling very guilty.

This guilt feeling grew as the days passed, I had been

signed off work for a week and during this time quite a few people from our church visited me. Most of them came with the intention of sympathizing and encouraging me. Few succeeded. I have since found that this is a common experience for those who have miscarriages.

A long-standing friend of mine, Jane, had married, as I did, whilst still at college. Her husband finished his degree and then went on to do a PhD, before going abroad on a one year contract, so it was some six years before they were settled and therefore able to have a family. Jane was one of the lucky ones, in that she fell pregnant after the second month and she, like us, was overjoyed that after such a long wait, albeit voluntary, she was going to be a mother.

One night, I answered the telephone and to my great surprise I heard her voice. It had been more than three years since we had seen each other and our letter writing was sporadic to say the least. We made polite conversation for a while and then, rather hesitantly she said, 'I do hope you don't mind my phoning you after all this time, but I just had to talk to you. Phil and I have just been through what you and Ian experienced.' For a moment my mind went completely blank and then, I knew. All I could say was 'Jane, I am so sorry.'

'Yes,' she replied, 'I knew you would be. That's why I rang you. People have been very kind but I just had to talk to someone who'd actually been through it. Someone who would understand.'

I knew exactly what she meant. Many people had visited me but the one who helped me the most was a lady in her late fifties, who came through the front door and put her arms around me; 'I lost two,' she said and together we cried. Later as we talked I was so receptive to her advice, because I knew that she had been through it too.

As Jane went on talking I relived our earlier experience. She told me how people had assured her that she was young yet, that she would soon be pregnant again, that this was a sign that all was well physically, that many women had early miscarriages and didn't even know it . . .

'I know all that and much more—in my head. It doesn't

help my feelings though does it? I feel so odd, kind of empty and wasted. Do you know what I mean?'

Again I knew. In the early weeks of pregnancy, and especially a first pregnancy, you are very aware of the miracle taking place within you. Throughout the day you find yourself thinking that within you there is life, new life, growing and developing, precious life. The sickness, the excessive tiredness, the slight muzziness and other individual symptoms experienced by women are a constant reminder of this special gift from God.

Then, after the miscarriage, it's all gone. Your body is 'back to normal', it is wholly yours again and it feels empty. For a little while you feel as though your body has no purpose any more. Another friend, Penny, told me years later:

'Having a miscarriage is like losing your child. From the moment you know you are pregnant, you begin to think about your baby—not the foetus. It's the child and then suddenly it's gone. If a child dies you grieve for it. You have a funeral service, people understand your need to grieve, they let you talk, they support you. After a miscarriage, people don't let you grieve. At first, you are allowed to cry and to talk, but then in a couple of weeks you are supposed to be normal and so it's locked away. You don't talk about it any more and you certainly aren't free to grieve.'

It was a new thought to me, but I began to see what she meant. Indeed, I have since heard that some women who are going through the emotional trauma of infertility, feel that menstruation is like the 'death' of a child, albeit a potential child. Personally, I never felt that way, although the time of menstruation is very depressing and fraught with emotion when you are waiting for a pregnancy.

A girl I met recently, Fiona, miscarried at twelve weeks. She was given ten days leave from work to recover, as much from the dilatation and curettage (D&C*) as from the miscarriage. At the end of that time she felt fine physically and was quite content to return to work. Two days later her boss sent her home. A small upset in the office had caused her, quite uncharacteristically, to burst into tears and having once begun she could not stop. She said to me, 'I felt such a fool'. But why should she? If she had lost a new-born baby, or a one-year-old everyone would have been aware that she would be vulnerable for some time. She would have been given room to grieve. Penny was right.

As Fiona and I talked she said, 'Of course, Peter has had it worse.' I asked her to explain. 'Well,' she replied, 'during the time that I was at home, people visited me, brought me flowers, stayed to chat. For at least ten days I was given the chance to unburden. But Peter was at work most of the time and in the evenings or at the weekend, people seemed to clam up when he was there, or totally ignored him. I suppose people didn't realise that he was disappointed as well.'

It is such a common misunderstanding, but quite natural. It is, after all, the woman who has been pregnant, she has the maternal feelings, she has had the physical discomfort. Obviously won't she be the most disappointed? What is more, most of the people who visit are women and they prefer to talk to the wife. Many of these ask extremely intimate details and the presence of the husband may be embarrassing.

However, many husbands feel like Ian and Peter did, especially if there has been any element of waiting. He, too, is aware that a life has been lost, flesh of his flesh; he knows that there will now be a delay, because most couples are advised to wait until the wife has had three normal menstrual cycles before trying again; and he is very concerned for his wife. A young girl, Jackie, was particularly aware of this:

'Gavin wasn't at all concerned about the baby. Frankly, he wasn't too fussed about having a family, as he felt that children would be a bit of an intrusion into our marriage and our pattern of living. But he was very upset for me. He said he wished that he could have been pregnant so that he could have had the pain and the D & C. He also wished that he could have taken my sadness and depression. That's what upset him most.'

Miscarriages are draining, physically, emotionally, and spiritually; but they can also be a time of learning. We went through a phase of depression and self-pity, but when we finally emerged we realized that we had grown closer to each other and to God. We were more dependant on Him than we had been and more willing to be guided by him.

As we tried to take stock objectively we realized that it had been a necessary step. I *had been* pregnant. For that we praised the Lord and began to look forward with hope.

Practical hints on how to cope with a miscarriage

1 As soon as you know what is happening ask yourself how badly you want this baby. If the answer is 'desperately', call your husband or a relative, then drop everything and go straight home. Call the doctor when you get in and then go to bed and stay there. That way you will know you did your best.
2 If at all possible get your husband to be with you when you see the doctor. It gives you moral support and it helps him to stay in the picture.
3 Don't be afraid of your feelings. It is natural to feel bereaved so let go and grieve for the baby you have lost, however early the miscarriage. Talk about it to someone who will understand.
4 Don't let your husband feel left out. He can't support you all the time, he too has to grieve. Help him to do so.
5 Your doctor will advise you to wait a while before trying again. Be positive about this enforced waiting time. Do something outrageous that you wouldn't be able to do if you were still pregnant—like skiing, underwater diving, hang gliding, a hiking holiday, six nights out on the trot,—anything fun and crazy that appeals to you both!
6 Tell God exactly how you feel. He will understand and you can let Him shoulder your disappointments and give you instead the peace you need.

3. Disillusionment: This Can't be Happening to Us

Why Us, Lord?

Why us, Lord?
Why can't we have children,
normally,
like other couples?
Why do we have to wait?

It's hard, you know,
Seeing all my friends get pregnant
have beautiful babies,
Even my sister, Lord,
I hardly call that fair.

Do you know how I feel?
I'll tell you.

I feel empty
bereft
unfulfilled
My arms ache
I have a pain inside
like growing pains
Except that I'm not growing.

I yearn, Lord, to have and to hold my own baby.

I am ashamed,
because I have not conceived
What is the point of this body
If it cannot function as it should?

I am a failure as a woman

You made me, Lord
You have allowed this to happen.
You
Give me
The strength to cope.

A year later, we were still waiting, but with less hope. It seemed to us that all our friends were being delivered of beautiful, bouncing babies. As time passed, our rejoicing in other people's happiness became tinged with sadness and envy and we began to dread the sight of the postman, for fear that he would bring another 'New Arrival' card!

We began to feel that every magazine, every newspaper, every television programme, every sermon, thrust before us pregnancy, babies or family life. We tried to keep a sense of humour and proportion, but it wasn't always easy. We had become very sensitive and although we knew that we were often touchy and unreasonable, we couldn't do a lot about it. Many people feel this way, female and male, married or single. The desire to have your own genetical child flesh of your flesh, can be as strong in a man as in a woman, or in a single person as in a married. It doesn't matter who you are or what your particular circumstances, if you have a deep inner longing to have a child then the ache of this thwarted desire is extremely painful.

Involuntary childlessness slowly corrodes away at your inner self, without you even noticing what is happening. Suddenly, we became aware that the *desire* to have a baby had become an *obsession*. I was totally absorbed by my monthly cycle, (which by now had become completely erratic), by other people's children and the way they behaved towards us.

We were filled with a hopeless longing and began to feel that everyone could see right through us. We over-reacted to harmless comments, thinking that they implied criticism or that they were veiled hints. However, though much was imaginary, there was a lot which was not. Never will I forget an occasion when we had a party of people from our old church drop by for the afternoon. During their stay a young mother proudly showed me her eighteen-month-old child, telling me all about her latest achievements. As she talked she pushed the child forward for me to hold.

I always had a struggle in a situation like this. I didn't want to be pacified by being given another mother's child and yet I longed to cuddle a baby. I was like a split personality, but in this instance, not wanting to offend I took the little girl.

Immediately she did exactly what I had dreaded. She began to protest, long and loud at being severed from her doting mother. I became self-conscious, unsure of how to quieten the child and yet aware that this was irrational. After watching my hopeless efforts the hovering mother took the child saying, 'You find it really hard to relate to children don't you?'

Having no children of our own made us very aware of other people's children, the way that they were brought up, discipline and so on. Like many other childless couples, we became very critical. Often we would come home and one or other would say, 'When we have a family we are not going to do that!'

Some friends, Alison and Mark, are just the same. Mark has no sperms and so they know that they cannot naturally have children of their own. Alison said, 'It has made us very critical of other parents. We really enjoy those families where the children are well disciplined and brought up, but Mark gets very angry against the parents of badly disciplined children. We become uncontrollably angry when we hear about children who are maltreated and also about women who have abortions. My sister-in-law frequently says to me, "If only you knew how awful it is to have four children, you wouldn't be worried about not having any of your own." I have absolutely no sympathy for her whatsoever!'

We too had friends complaining to us about the

difficulties of parenthood, the sleepless nights, the tantrums, the endless demands. How could we sympathise when we would have given almost anything to be coping with those very problems?

Every couple reacts to the experience of childlessness in a different way. A few accept it with comparative ease and look for positive outlets; others first have to go through a very dark passage; most have a feeling of shock and disbelief that this thing could happen to them. Infertility[2] is something which happens to someone else.

Whatever the reaction, however, some of the distress that is felt is a direct result of society's pressure and of well-meaning but tactless friends. Recently a lady talked with me about the infertility of some mutual friends. She said, 'I told them not to worry. I mean, after all, as I said to them, you could always go to the mission field. It's better not to have children when you're a missionary.'

Comments such as these show a total lack of understanding of what the couple are feeling and experiencing. At that time we were both over-sensitive, but I was particularly quick to react to thoughtless comments, and allowed them to fester in my mind to such an extent that sometimes I would feel unwilling to encounter that person again. Another couple, Sue and John had a three year wait before their first daughter was born and during that time Sue suffered from severe depression. She admitted to me, 'It was an awfully traumatic time. There seemed to be a total lack of understanding amongst our friends and there is no doubt in my mind that it is the woman who is hit the worst. You get so broody!'

So often in the past I had joked about being broody, but it was only at this time that I began to understand what it really meant. 'Broody' in the literal sense means a hen that is wanting to hatch chicks. It is now an accepted word, in the figurative sense and is defined in the Oxford Dictionary as 'feeling depressed'. I would put it much stronger than that. It is not depression from just any cause, but from the desire to have a baby. Being broody isn't just seeing a tiny baby and suddenly, fleetingly, thinking it might be nice to have one like it. To be really broody is to ache with a deep-rooted longing for a child of your own. It is to yearn physically for a baby to hold. It is to feel bereft, empty, unfulfilled.

Many women suffer from this, whether they are involuntarily childless, voluntarily childless or single. Kate is a friend of mine who was born to be a mother. She and Jonathon were married three years ago and moved to London, where Jonathon had a job with a large organization. He had at least two years training ahead and so Kate took a job in teaching and they bought a flat. Due to unforseeable circumstances the training has taken double the time and the mortgage commitments are greater than expected. Kate and Jonathon have chosen to remain childless until he has finished training and then they will move to a cheaper area.

'I'm living for that time,' says Kate. 'Sometimes I get so broody I don't know what to do with myself. My arms ache to hold a baby, there is a pain somewhere inside me gnawing away so that all day I seem to be thinking about it. During these black times I only seem to see pregnant women, newborn babies, overflowing prams. Most of my friends have had babies and at this time they usually want a babysitter!'

'When I am not broody, my desire for a baby is controlled, I have God's peace, but once I am in the throes of an attack all that is lost. I become hurt and bitter at the waiting, angry at no-one in particular and I cry a lot. It also hinders our love-making as I am often filled with an all-embracing sadness that yet again we will not produce a baby.'

How does she cope, knowing that her situation is one of choice? 'I remind myself that God has a reason for delaying our plans and I try to think positively about what I am learning—like patience! I also remind myself that Jonathon is almost as keen as I am to have a baby and that he, too, gets frustrated, so I try not to moan to him too much. Often I go out and buy one of the monthly magazines on motherhood and babies and indulge in a good session of baby-worship. It helps to accept your feelings and deal with them.'

Kate has all my admiration for dealing openly and

honestly with her desires. She is a wonderful babysitter and selflessly gives her time to parents who need a break from their demanding offspring. She uses her talents constructively, to the benefit of all. But there is ultimately a difference, as her situation is due to choice. For those who have no choice, either through infertility or through being single, to be involved with other people's children can bring heartache of its own, because at the end of the day, the child is not yours. It has to go back to its mother.

I well recall a young couple bringing their four-month-old baby to stay with us for a week-end. The mother, in genuine love and concern for me, shared her baby freely. During their stay I changed her, bathed her, fed her, rocked her to sleep and cuddled her at every available moment. The parents were totally selfless about their still-new baby. However, neither they nor I were to know how I was to suffer when they went home. Suddenly, the baby had gone and I was left with a faint aroma of dirty nappies, baby powder and sour milk—that and a gaping void. Never had I experienced anything as fierce as the longing to have and to hold my own child. I ached as hard as if I had lost my own baby. Through this I learnt a salutary lesson: never to allow another woman's baby to temporarily fill the place of our own.

Indeed, I never made that mistake again, but I made another. When, some years later a childless friend came to stay with me, just after we had our baby, I overprotected her.

I was so frightened that she would experience the same feelings, that I didn't encourage her to take part in the nappy-changing routine, the bathing and all the other baby-orientated tasks. When she left at the end of the week-end we suddenly realized that she hadn't held the baby once. That was just as big a mistake.

Each woman has to find out for herself whether having another woman's baby on a temporary basis is a help or hindrance to her. No matter what bonds of love form, or the responsibility, care and upbringing you share, the child belongs to someone else. The 'universal aunt', childminder, teacher, playgroup helper and so on all know that the child is 'on loan'.

Alison was born to be a mother and now that she and her husband have adopted two little boys, she takes her commitment very seriously. She is totally absorbed in and dedicated to the upbringing of her sons and it is obvious that she has a deep love for her children. Nevertheless, she admitted to me that it would have been a hindrance to have someone else's baby on a short-term basis. 'I could never have fostered,' she said, 'whether it was short-term or long-term. I become too involved and too attached, so that I could never give them up. Each time a foster child was taken from me, for whatever reason, I would have been heart-broken and I would have spent countless hours worrying about what was happening to them and whether they were being ill-treated.'

We each need to find out how much we, personally, can take and not be ashamed to accept our limitations. Society exerts great pressures and expectations and often it is easier to conform. Many people feel that if a couple really want children then adoption or fostering is the natural solution. In fact, in a report published by the Free Church Federal Council and The British Council of Churches[3], it is suggested that this solution might be recommended to couples before they consider medical intervention. This is a total misunderstanding of many of the emotions felt by the infertile couple.

We are whole people, physical, emotional, spiritual and in trying to find a solution to the problem of infertility, we must take all these three into account. When a couple first realize that they are having trouble conceiving, their primary reaction is one of shock, and usually they close their minds to the possibility that something might be wrong. Long before they decide to investigate the physical problems, they are having emotional and often spiritual problems. In Sue's words, 'Infertility will make or break a marriage'. Adoption or fostering is something you come to in time, when you have sorted out these problems.

It is not only the wife who suffers, although undoubtedly she is more deeply involved. During our year of waiting after that first miscarriage, Ian had his fair share of hurting and longing. At first we didn't realize what was happening, but at last I came out of my shell for long enough to see what was going on.Suddenly I was aware that Ian was avoiding swimming pools, parks, playgrounds and Saturday shopping. He couldn't stand the sight of fathers playing with their children or carrying them in a papoose. When at last I did get pregnant this was really brought home to me. We would be walking through a busy shopping centre, when Ian would nudge me and say, 'Look, over there, we'll soon have one like that.' Intent on my shopping list I would not have noticed the baby at all and I would find that in almost every case it was a father with a child that had caught his attention.

However, even when we realised what was happening, we did not talk about it very much to other people. It's not macho for men to have 'maternal' feelings. It's not British to let the stiff upper lip tremble. It's not christian to admit to feelings of despair or anger. So Ian hid his hurt, suppressed his longings, not talking about it except on rare occasions in the privacy of our home. Even then, he was so intent on supporting me, on upholding and encouraging my spirits that often he did not tell me how he felt.

Sue told me how John had been a tower of strength, listening to her, praying with her and for her, often until the early hours. Yet his own distress would finally show through when, on occasions, he would find that he was unable to make love to her. It was one of the few times that she was aware that he too was deeply upset by their problems.

Irrational anger is often a sign of inner turmoil and Alison would know that Mark was upset about their situation, when he let rip about some unsuspecting parent. Ian would often become extremely heated about lack of service or quality. The number of shop assistants who had faulty goods returned to them forcibly, is past counting! My docile husband, who could not normally be bothered to make a great song and dance about anything was slowly becoming aggressive.

During the second year Ian also became an avid squash player. At first I thought it was to do with keeping fit and young, but having watched him beat a ball about the court, during a practice session, I soon realised it had a greater therapeutic value than we thought, and I began to join him on the court!

Fertility problems can cause all manner of side-effects, apparent or not. Katherine Hall in her recently published book, Learning To Cope With Childlessness, writes, 'Doctors, psychiatrists, ministers and anyone who has acted simply as a listener to a friend in distress will all attest the destructive power of childlessness, an anguish which, concealed from the world in general, will manifest itself in all manner of physical or mental disorder, whose true cause is not always recognised even by the sufferer.'[4]

There always has to be a scapegoat to release inner tensions. Derek and Mandy have been trying for a family for eighteen months and are just beginning the long medical investigations. The strain is beginning to show. A few months ago all was well at work for both of them, but recently things have changed. Derek particularly is having many problems with his job. There are personal clashes and disagreements with other members of staff that have come as a complete surprise. His inner turmoil is creating a dissatisfaction with the job and he is unleashing some of his anger on his employees.

His life-style is being threatened by their failure to have children so far and it is spilling over not only into his work but also into his church life. He feels that his manhood is being threatened and therefore is needing to be reassured and to somehow 'prove' his maleness. He is becoming increasingly dogmatic and unreasonable, refusing to accept that his views might not be the only right ones. He is not alone in this. Most men feel that their manhood is threatened, at least until the reason for their childlessness as a couple is discovered. An article in Newsweek[5] quotes a husband with fertility problems as saying, 'There is nothing that hits into the very essence of what I am as a man more than this.' Some continue to feel that way, even if the problem lies with the wife, because of the pressures of society.

Abraham obviously suffered from social pressures and

his distress that Sarah could not give him a child is clearly shown in Genesis 15. 1 - 3.

'After this the word of the Lord came to Abram in a vision; Do not be afraid, Abram,
I am your shield,
your very great reward.'

> But Abram said, "O Sovereign Lord, what can you give me since I remain childless and the one who will inherit my estate is Eliezer of Damascus? so a servant in my household will be my heir." '(NIV)

Could this godly man really feel this way? That all God's blessings were useless, as nothing, simply because he was deprived of children. Yes, a godly man can feel thus. Many will say that in Abraham's day children, more particularly sons, were essential and that the Jews live through their sons after death. Therefore, if they are childless there will be no afterlife. Some say that it is the same in the East today, but not in the West, that there is no social stigma about not having children. Don't you believe it!

Children are very important. If you want a child, then the inability to have one is heartbreaking and the lack of a family seems to put you in a different social strata. In Christian circles the stigma seems to be emphasized even more, as stress is laid on the God-created *family* structure.

In 'Choices of Childlessness'[4], the authors state that 'In much of our society it is socially unacceptable for a couple to be childless. Expectations about infertility are widespread . . . Such expectations are very strong and can have powerful effects on those who fail to fulfill them.' They acknowledge the pressures of society and later, they emphasize the Christian point of view;

> 'procreation of children . . . may seem as a special expression of the faith that the future is not to be determined by the powers of this world, and by the power of the crucified and risen Son of God. Children are a symbol of hope. They may appear to be hostages to fortune, but Christians see them as in fact pledges of the love and fidelity of God.

> This significance of children for the Christian community has been expressed as follows: "There is much that could be done that might be considered more important than having children. Children take time and energy, psychologically and physically, that prevents us from being better scholars, important businessmen , serving the poor or attacking the structures of injustice. But it is the Christian's claim that God's kingdom is not to be built by us, that gives us the patience, in a world of injustice, to insist that nothing is more important than having and rearing children. We do this not because we hope our children will choose to be the next generation of those who carry the story of God in the world. We must remember that our hope is not in our children but in the God who gives us and them grounds of hope." '

For Christians, children are one of the highest vocational callings and as such, childlessness within the Christian community is even harder to accept.

We, for one, felt this very acutely and began to wonder whether emigration might not be a happy solution! Sue and John and Paul and Louisa were particularly vulnerable as they are both in the full time ministry.

In Paul and Louisa's case their problems had been shared with the elders fairly early on, because of the kind of questions that were being asked. They found people generally sympathetic and caring, but their private lives were no longer private. Everyone was watching and waiting and one of the worst things to cope with was blatant pity.

They told me that it was difficult dealing with family problems for a variety of reasons. It was a sensitive area in their lives and so it was hard to listen to whining parents complaining about their responsibilities. How do you help a couple with unwanted children, who are disinterested in them? What of the single mother? What do you say to the sixteen year old who has accidentally got pregnant? How do you sympathize with the woman who has guilt feelings about an abortion? It is only God who can give the grace to be loving and compassionate in situations such as these.

Sue and John told me of a different problem. They were in a church where they were the youngest couple and in a situation where they could not share their problems with the elders. They found that they were continually misunderstood and that members of the church made reference to their lack of a family. They felt that their work was hampered by this and that some of the members considered them unqualified in some respects. A bit like the single pastor.

Being childless can cause you to become introspective. You begin to lose your self-esteem and your self-confidence. You begin to lose the ability to communicate satisfactorily at a normal level.

Breaking point, for us, finally came when first my best-friend and then my newly-wed sister, both became pregnant. Both found it difficult to tell us. My friend, who had moved away to New Zealand, took three months to find the words and finally wrote a lengthy, apologetic letter. My sister decided not to phone but write. The letter was tear-stained and it was then that we really became aware that people did not know how to handle our situation.

Anger, hurt, frustration, jealousy, self-pity washed over us. We gave up pretending to ourselves that we could cope and yelled at the Lord. We had begged Him not to let these two things happen to us. So *why*? Didn't He promise that He wouldn't try us beyond our capabilities?

We were in a tunnel of darkness so long that we couldn't see the light at the end. God made us and gave us our natural desire for a child. It seemed as though our marriage had no pivot, we were incomplete; a jigsaw with pieces missing. In her book, Katherine Hall writes about this lack of fulfilment,

> '(1 Sam. 1.6) Hannah's yearning for a child was so intense that she promised him to the Lord even before he was born . . . What then was the point of having a child only to give him away? The answer presumably lies in the basic God-given need of a

husband and wife for fulfilment in their marriage, for the child who sets the seal on their union and renders it fruitful. Even if the child Samuel's parents hardly saw him again, he was indubitably there, the object of love and prayer and thought even in his absence. He was the focus for their marriage.'[6]

We had reached that sense of pointlessness; all the pent-up emotions, fears and hang-ups of the last months surged to the fore, threatening to envelop us. We were both filled with feelings of inadequacy; I felt less than female, Ian felt a failure as a man.

Most couples have this sense of personal failure. Sue put it to me this way: 'I just didn't feel like a woman. I felt that my body was useless and that it wouldn't function properly. As the months went by I came to despise my body. I felt naked and insecure, as though everyone could see everything that was going on inside me. I couldn't bear to see myself naked in a mirror and I didn't want John to touch me at all. My body was an abomination to me.'

Sue felt this way despite the fact that the problem was not all on her side. It was in fact fifty-fifty, because they both had too high a prolactin level, Sue was not ovulating and John had a very low sperm count. Inevitably many of the emotions are focused around the body, because pregnancy changes a woman's body. It is easy to become obsessed about weight, for example. Some women allow themselves to get fat, others become determined to stay post-card thin. Most women, at some time, experience the feeling that they do not want to be touched and some men go through temporary impotence.

We were very aware of these feelings and because we felt inadequate and insecure we began to question God's will. Was it really in His plan for us to remain childless? Should we throw ourselves into our careers and our church life? Would He allow us to have children by adoption or fostering? Was it going against God's will to seek medical advice and how far could we go with medical aid? Should we, like the widow (Luke 18.8), badger God to change His mind? Could we change His will?

We thrashed around each question, desperately seeking coherent answers. Those christians whom we had the courage to question, merely offered platitudes or startlingly naive advice. One dear Christian lady said to us, 'Well, of course, I know what your problem is, you're being too scientific. Throw away your temperature charts, just relax and love each other. You'll get pregnant immediately. That's what God intends.' We began to feel very isolated.

At last I did what I should have done at the very beginning, I opened my Bible. To my utter astonishment, I discovered that there are at least seven women in the Bible, who are mentioned in connection with their infertility; Sarah (Genesis 16, 18, 25), Rebekah (Genesis 25), Rachel (Genesis 30), Manoah's wife (Judges 13), Hannah (1 Sam 1), the Shunamite (2 Kings 4) and Elizabeth (Luke 1).

As I read each story, some of the anger and desolation flowed out of me as each woman reached out to comfort me. Each had something to say to me and in time I was to learn from them all, but at this particular time it was Sarah and Hannah who really helped me.

Sarah, the wife of Abraham had borne him no children and this carried a terrible social stigma. It was considered to be the duty of the wife to provide her husband with children, and more particularly with sons. Failure to do so was automatically assumed to be the fault of the woman and therefore, she had failed in her duty. This meant that the husband had the right to go and obtain an heir by another woman.

It is the same in some countries in the East, today. A missionary couple wrote to me to tell of their experiences of infertility. One of the particular problems they faced was the severe attitude of local people where they live, where a woman could be thrown out and left homeless if she failed to produce a child for her husband. It has given them a deep desire as a couple to use their experience of childlessness to enable them to help couples and especially women who face this problem.

Sarah had failed in her duty to Abraham and so she provided her husband with her maidservant, so that she might have a child 'by proxy'. In effect, Hagar became a surrogate mother.

> 'Abram slept with Hagar and she conceived. When she knew she was pregnant, she began to despise her mistress. Then Sarah said to Abram, "You are responsible for the wrong I am suffering. I put my servant in your arms and now that she knows she is pregnant, she despises me. May the Lord judge between you and me" ' (Genesis 16. 4,5,NIV).

How human she is in her display of irrational anger! How often I have been filled with unreasonable anger, which I have taken out on my innocent husband! I could identify with Sarah.

> 'Then the Lord said, "I will surely return to you about this time next year and Sarah your wife will have a son." Now Sarah was listening at the entrance to the tent, which was behind him. Abraham and Sarah were already old and well advanced in years and Sarah was past the age of childbearing. So Sarah laughed to herself as she thought, "After I am worn out and my master is old, will I now have this pleasure?" ' (Genesis 18. 10-12,NIV)

Nowadays Sarah would be described as an elderly primagravida and the doctors would shake their heads over the outcome of such a late pregnancy. Sarah was physically past it and had long given up hoping. It is no wonder that she should laugh and question whether the angelic visitors had delivered the right message. However, when the miracle does in fact happen, she is quick to repent and to give God all the glory.

> 'Now the Lord was gracious to Sarah . . . and . . . did for Sarah what he had promised . . . Abraham gave the name Isaac to the son Sarah bore him . . . Sarah said "God has brought me laughter, and everyone who hears about this will laugh with me" ' (Genesis 21 1-6 NIV).

Sarah brings hope to those who are past hope and so does Hannah. How I wish I could have talked to her! It is Hannah who shows all the grief, crying endlessly, refusing food, losing her perspective. Would she, I wonder, be one of the babysnatchers today? This tormented lady knew the deep physical yearning, the total obsession with having a child, the shame, the anger, the despair.

> ' . . . the Lord had closed (Hannah's) womb. And because the Lord had closed her womb, her rival kept provoking her in order to irritate her. This went on year after year. Whenever Hannah went up to the house of the Lord, her rival provoked her till she wept and would not eat. Elkanah her husband would say to her, "Hannah, why are you weeping? Why don't you eat? Don't I mean more to you than 10 sons?"
> . . . In bitterness of soul Hannah wept much and prayed to the Lord. And she made a vow saying, "O Lord Almighty, if you will only look upon your servant's misery and remember me, and not forget your servant but give her a son, then I will give him to the Lord for all the days of his life, and no razor will ever be used on his head."
> As she kept on praying to the Lord, Eli (the priest) observed her mouth. Hannah was praying in her heart and her lips were moving but her voice was not heard. Eli thought she was drunk . . . .
> "Not so, my lord," Hannah replied, "I am a woman who is deeply troubled. I have not been drinking wine or beer; I was pouring out my soul to the Lord. Do not take your servant for a wicked woman; I have been praying here out of my great anguish and grief."
> Eli answered, "Go in peace, and may the God of Israel grant you what you have asked of him." . . . .
> So in the course of time Hannah conceived and gave birth to a son. She named him Samuel, saying, "Because I asked the Lord for Him." ' (1 Sam 1. 5-17, 20)

Here was a woman who was desperate enough to bargain with God and how many of us have been tempted to do that? Here was a woman who was so grief-stricken that the priest thought she was drunk. Here was a woman obsessed with having a baby. I saw a self-portrait.

Practical hints on dealing with broodiness

1 Learn to recognize the early signs of broodiness so that you can take action before you get too depressed.
2 Try not to be alone too much. Talk about the way you feel to your husband or someone else who understands. Do explain to your husband how you feel and try to make him see that your desire for children is not a reflection on your personal relationship. He might not experience your feelings in depth but it will help him to understand and to support you.
3 Go out and do something for someone else. This will help to improve your sense of self-worth.
4 Know what makes you particularly upset, e.g. newborn babies, pregnant ladies, baby dolls and avoid them until the worst of it is over.
5 Do something you enjoy—preferably something that will absorb your mind and tire you out.
6 Read the story of Hannah in 1 Samuel 1. Talk to the Lord about the way you feel. Hannah did.
7 Get plenty of sleep. Self-pity and depression are at their worst if you are over-tired.
8 Remember that broodiness is often related to the menstrual cycle. So be encouraged because it will take its natural course and then pass!

4. Investigation: Tests, More Tests and Treatment

The Hospital

I am sick of grey walls
Narrow corridors
White coats.

I am tired of probing questions
Endless tests
Marking time

Another face
Another opinion
Another wait
And see

Why did I ever start

I am just
another case history

Another faceless name
Another unsolved problem

Short staffed
Hard up

Regimented
Daily grind
How can they understand
They are doing their best

In time
A diagnosis
Inconclusive

Here in this germ-free sterile ward
They say that I am not sterile.

There is a chance
A hope
A future

Wait and see.

We finally embarked on the medical merry-go-round. This is just as dizzying as it sounds and is only for the very determined. You need a shield of stainless steel, the persistence of a pneumatic drill and the strength of Concorde to break barriers, for in general, there is a lethargic lack of interest in the problem.

Ian and I had talked at length about our situation and had come to the conclusion that there were no major obstacles to our seeking medical aid. We had certainly not received any guidance which would lead to us remaining childless, in order to follow a certain vocation. In fact, we both felt quite strongly that we should do everything possible to become parents, whether of our own children or through adopting or fostering.

When we visited our GP, she was somewhat pessimistic about the chances of getting an appointment at the local infertility clinic. Like so many doctors who shrug their overburdened shoulders, she recommended us, quite kindly to relax and keep trying. Infertility clinics are few and far between and so they usually have long waiting lists. She estimated that we would wait at least six months before we got an appointment, which only served to increase our desire to be put on the waiting list!

The Lord sorted out the timing for us and we did in fact get an appointment within a month. When we got that prized appointment, our hopes soared and we began to see life much more positively. This seemed to us like the gateway to success, but we were to be rudely awoken.

On the morning of the appointment I woke up with mixed feelings. I was excited and hopeful, but I was also scared and apprehensive. Although I had actually worked in the hospital for a while I had never been near the maternity wing. The corridor stretched endlessly before us but we soon passed into an annexe, which seemed like the back of beyond.

We came to a large reception desk and I assumed we had taken a wrong turning. We were surrounded by heavily pregnant women, all milling around having their weights checked or handing in urine samples. We were just beginning to back off when the nurse at the desk spotted us and asked what we wanted.

Reluctantly we approached the desk and silently handed her our appointment letter. She scanned it, handed me a bottle for a urine test and told Ian to take a seat. As I headed for the toilet, I idly wondered whether she thought I was in the early weeks of pregnancy!

By the time I returned to Ian he was sitting stiffly on a chair in the farthest corner of the room, a tense look about his mouth. I took the seat next to his and surveyed the room. Every stage of pregnancy was graphically illustrated before us. Women of every size and shape, many with tiresome toddlers demanding their wearied attention, talking animatedly about their latest symptom or bemoaning their fate. The walls were liberally covered with posters giving advice to the pregnant mother and warning her against the dangers that might befall her, if she smoked excessively or lifted heavy objects the wrong way.

Idly I opened the book I had brought with me, but my concentration was elsewhere. My insides were churning like a butter making machine and my ears were straining to catch the names being called out over the tannoy system. Even now I can capture again the vision, the smell and the deafening noise of that waiting room.

At last we were called and we made our way into the narrow corridor, rapidly reading the door names, until at last we found the correct consulting room. Through a member of the family, we were privileged enough to see the consultant at our first appointment. However, we were not prepared to find another doctor, two students and a nurse also waiting for us. It was a large London teaching hospital and we learned that students were frequently present at interviews.

The consultant began a detailed and intimate questioning that we answered as positively as posible. 'How old are you? How long have you been married? How long have you been trying for a family?' No problems there. 'Have either of you ever had a child by another person?' Mutely we shook our heads. He glanced from one to the other of us and rephrased his question, 'Have either of you ever been married before?' Again we shook our heads and Ian said 'No'.

There was an uncomfortable movement from one of the students which seemed to trigger the Consultant, who said apologetically, 'I'm sorry I have to ask these questions, but if either of you had ever had a child it would simplify things. You see, we could then rule out one of you as being infertile.'

The questions went on, delving into the frequency and satisfaction of our sex lives and finally moving into a more practical phase. Eagerly I handed him my temperature charts. He glanced at them and roared with laughter before handing them to the other doctor. 'You're a textbook case, my dear,' he said nodding at the smile on the other man's face. He took the charts back and handed them to the students. 'I've never seen such good ovulation graphs! In fact, I'd like to keep them for my tutorials.' I was waiting for him to ask what textbook I'd used.

He kept the charts and then ushered me behind a green curtain for a medical examination. As I got dressed again afterwards I could hear him asking more detailed questions of my husband and was glad of the short respite.

The consultation was over. He said that as far as he

could see there was nothing wrong. However, he suggested that Ian should have a semen analysis done and that I should have a laparoscopy.* There was no mention of blood tests or any other test. Then he said, 'You may have to wait some time for the laparoscopy, but that's all to the good. You will probably get pregnant before that happens. We don't really know what part the brain plays in conception, but we do believe that it has a definite effect. If you are very worried about something or under a lot of stress, we think it might hinder the natural processes. The best advice I can give you at this moment is to go home, relax and take things as they come. You haven't really been trying very long and you're young yet. Try not to be too intense and you'll find you conceive unexpectedly. It often happens.'

We were out in the busy main road and hurrying towards our car before either of us spoke. Ian slipped his arm around me and I burst out, 'It would seem that we are psychological cases!' Ian laughed, in his opinion it was the doctor's usual let-out clause when he could think of no other cause. His only reply to me was, 'I don't like having an audience!' That was one of the drawbacks of a teaching hospital and later we found many more.

In the following three months we did try to take life a little more quietly. I tried to keep my mind off having a baby, but it was very difficult when we were ruled by the temperature charts. My first thought in the morning was inevitably related to this subject, as I would roll over to turn the alarm clock off and pick up the thermometer in one movement. My turn to fall asleep again, until Ian removed the thermometer and nudged me awake to take a mug of tea. Record the reading on the graph and glance to see whether it was the right time of the month.

As we approached the 'fertile period' we had been told to abstain from love-making for three days prior to the expected temperature rise. Then we were to have intercourse on the day of the temperature rise, not the next day, but the one after that. Wedlock had become wedclock and it didn't make for a relaxed approach.

Our local GP had given us her own brand of advice. 'Work out from your charts when you are most likely to be fertile, then keep several evenings free around that time. When your temperature rises, ring your best friends and invite them round to a fertility party. Have a good meal, plenty of wine and relax in the company of good friends. Then send them home early and go to bed. It usually works!'

I did keep the diary free and we did have a relaxed dinner for two. Maybe it was the convivial company that was missing! Anyway we enjoyed ourselves and I suppose that is half the secret.

Eventually I went in to have my laparoscopy done. The day started badly for me, because I had been told to arrive at 9 am ready for the operation that afternoon. We arrived on time and hung around for about an hour, when we were told that the operating list was for the next day and so I had another thirty-six hours to wait. However, they managed to keep me busy. During the morning I had blood samples taken from me by a young doctor who chatted cheerfully about the procedure.

He explained that a laparoscopy is a very simple operation. It is almost always done under general anaesthetic and its real value is that it allows the surgeon to investigate in detail the woman's ovaries and Fallopian tubes and in some cases to carry out minor surgery. It can often prevent major surgery later on and is a very safe procedure (less than 2 in 100 women suffer any complications[9]).

The procedure is to put carbon dioxide gas into the abdominal cavity via a needle inserted at the umbilicus. This acts in such a way as to blow out the organs so that the surgeon has better visibility. A one-inch-long incision is then made at the navel and a laparoscope is inserted through it. This is a long thin instrument like a telescope. The surgeon then takes a good look around. In many cases a dye is put into the inflated cavity, through the cervix. The dye should travel up the Fallopian tubes and should come out of the ends, providing there are no blockages. Tubal abnormalities represent about 25% of all causes of female infertility[10] and the number of women who are infertile because of blocked tubes is rising. It is one of the easiest conditions to diagnose, although about the most difficult to cure!

During the afternoon my parents came across London to visit me and help while away the hours. I was so grateful to them because I was already clock-watching. In the middle of this I was called away by another doctor. More blood tests, because they had lost the ones taken that morning.

I was beginning to feel less than confident by the time the anaesthetist appeared the next morning. 'Mrs Cooke?', she queried and then rifled frantically through her notes. At last she heaved a sigh of relief, 'I thought we'd lost your notes, but here they are.' I hoped they would not lose them later on, because the lady before me was an abortion and the lady after me a sterilisation. I did not want to get muddled up with either of them!

As we prepared for the operations we were to undergo, we chatted freely. The fact that we were all rather nervous and uncertain about the outcome, meant that we dropped the cool British reserve amd talked openly and honestly. Some of the talk did not help me. The lady with the sterilisation was voluble to say the least and told anyone who would listen that she already had two children and that she simply couldn't bear to have any more. Children were a menace, she'd done her duty and she was not going to run the risk that she might have any more. One brave patient suggested that she might regret that decision if she were to be widowed. She replied nonchalantly that she could always get it reversed.

I tried not to listen as she went off to talk to someone else, only to discover that the patient having an abortion was being questioned by the same brave spokesman. She was a young girl, not quite twenty, it had been an accident and she did not want the baby. She was applauded by her examiner, who turned out to be having a hysterectomy, and I buried my nose in a book, terrified that she would ask me my medical history.

By the time I came to go to theatre, I was scared out of my wits and ashamed of my feelings. Not only was I a Christian, but I had worked in a hospital, this hospital. Therein lay part of the problem, because I could not rid my mind of some of the medical accidents I had seen.

Again and again I reminded myself that the percentage of errors was minute. Again and again I prayed and read my Bible begging the Lord to give me peace. He is ever present and He does.

The anaesthetist was very relaxed and chatted quietly to me. My smiles were rather forced and my mouth dry, but I didn't have long to be social. As the anaesthetic flowed into me I sank thankfully and most willingly into oblivion.

My first conscious awareness was of a female voice urging me to wake up. I was forced into the sitting up position, but felt so violently sick that the hands instantly returned me to the horizontal position! My next memory is of being made to wash my hands and face. A voice which seemed to jar on my ears commented that I was still out for the count and suggested I skip supper and sleep it off. I mentally applauded her perception, sinking gratefully into sleep once more.

Ian's visit was lost in brief moments of awareness, followed by long silences as I slept again before dragging myself back to the present. He told me later that he didn't get two coherent words from me the whole time he sat there, which I have since understood is quite common.

Next day, awake at last and refreshed from a shower and some breakfast, I sat on my bed watching yet another doctor do his rounds, discharging patients and telling them the outcome of their operation. He seemed to be moving so slowly. Finally, the unknown face gazed at me over my medical notes and said, 'Well, Mrs Cooke, you have one blocked Fallopian tube, but the other one is clear. You can go home as soon as you are ready.'

I swallowed hard, focused on his white overall and asked, 'Does that mean that I only have a fifty-fifty chance of getting pregnant?'

He closed my notes and shook his head, 'No, it's not as clear cut as that. It does reduce your chances but not fifty-fifty. All you need is one egg and one tube. The ovaries don't always produce eggs alternately and even if they did the Fallopian tubes can 'wave around' and so the good one could catch the egg, whichever ovary produced it. Providing your husband is alright there is nothing to worry about.'

'And is he?'

'I don't know. I'm afraid we've lost the results, so he'll have to repeat the test. I'll make a note for you to return in three months, to get the results and have a check-up. By then you'll probably be pregnant.' He grinned, wished me good day and moved on.

I was glad to be home, glad that the doctor had found something but disappointed that there was nothing to be done. Just more waiting. We were both cross that they had lost Ian's results and I did feel that to operate on me without knowing whether Ian was alright, was a bit premature—even though I was glad that they had found the blocked tube. My thoughts were rather muddled, but in general I was disappointed at the outcome. Waiting, more waiting and I was short on patience.

We returned in the allotted time, still not pregnant and saw yet another doctor. This time they had the results and they told us that Ian had a lower-than-average sperm count. They did not give us the figures and we were too naive to ask. The doctor simply told us that it was still possible to get pregnant.

There are several different things that are investigated during a sperm analysis such as the volume, sperm count, sperm motility, normality of the specimen and its chemical make-up.

In Ian's case the doctor only mentioned the sperm count and he didn't seem to be worried about that. Nevertheless it has been said that a subtle problem in the husband and a subtle problem in the wife makes for one major fertility problem.

An appointment was made for us to return to the hospital one year later if I was still not pregnant. Apart from that we heard the usual platitudes and assurances, before taking ourselves off fast. Although it was to be another year and a half and many more tests and treatments, we never returned to that hospital.

Our morale nose-dived at this point. The medical profession had made a token gesture and now we had to get on with it. There were numerous tests that had not been carried out, but we did know that there was something wrong with both of us and that it was a waiting game we were playing. It was a small comfort to know that both of us had a problem and that neither was 'to blame', yet we had new disappointments and frustrations.

Up until now it had been a question of 'Why can't we get pregnant, what's wrong with whom?' Now we knew and yet we were no better off. The strain of the medical tests, the endless frustrations and the promise of more waiting, began to erode our marriage relationship.

What couple can honestly say that they have never, even for a split second, wondered whether their marriage was a mistake (and that does not only apply to those of us who suffer fertility problems). It is so easy to think 'if only'. Ian could have looked at me and thought 'I have a low sperm count but if she didn't have a blocked fallopian tube we could have a baby.' I, too, could have blamed Ian for reducing my chances.

In moments of depression it is so easy to apportion blame. It is in a way a release so that you don't have to carry the responsibility. A boxer practises by hitting a punchbag. What a useful installation in the spare bedroom that would have been, so that in moments of depression, anger or frustration we could have punched the life out of it.

It might have saved the niggling doubts that crept in. 'She wants a baby so much—is it more important to her than our love?' Or maybe the feeling of guilt, 'If I hadn't got a low sperm count, she could have a baby. I have brought her such a burden of grief.'

Ian was a tower of strength to me and I remember him assuring me that our love and our marriage were more important to him than a family. Unlike Elkanah (I Samuel 1.8), I never had to ask the question, 'Am I not more to you than ten sons?' We held on to our love for each other and tried not to be impatient. For a little while, we abandoned medical intervention.

Another couple who were fortunate enough to live in an area where there was a proper infertility clinic are Sue and John. They had been to their own GP who was singularly uninterested in their problems and always anxious to get on to the next patient. Sue badgered him constantly, until in desperation to be rid of her, he referred them to the clinic. From that moment on Sue found that the medical profession was extremely helpful, understanding and sympathetic.

Sue was given every medical test and finally a laparoscopy, so that she was confident that the final diagnosis was comprehensive. John's sperm count was found to be so low that they did not hold much hope and in addition Sue had very low hormone levels. She was given treatment for this, but without much hope and at this point God intervened. Sue and John were desperate for a child and very distressed by the results of the medical investigations. They had no choice left but to pray for a miracle, and the Lord in His goodness granted their wish. Miraculously within six months Sue was pregnant and they had a beautiful daughter. But then, when they tried for their second child it started all over again. Sue said, 'It is much, much worse the second time round, because you know a little bit about what you are going to go through. You wonder if you can bear all the trauma, stress and waiting all over again. It is also harder because you are older.'

Nevertheless they did go through it again. More medical facts were brought to light and the doctors admitted that they did not know how she had achieved one pregnancy. Sue was not ovulating at all, in addition to the low hormone level.

John had a very high prolactin level, which is thought to decrease sperm formation.* He was given the drug Bromocriptine,* but he was so violently sick that he had to stop taking it. Later he discovered that taking it with food often helps to repress the sickness.

Once more Sue was given hormone treatment. Among other things she was put on Clomid,* which stimulates ovulation in 70-80% of women. In about 13% of cases it causes multiple births, but these are usually twins. The other drug frequently used to stimulate ovulation is Pergonal,* which must be very carefully controlled if it is not to produce multiple pregnancies, often triplets or more.

Sue and John are grateful to the medical profession,

who were honest with them and admitted that they did not think their chances were very high for a second pregnancy. When John had to stop taking the Bromocriptine, everyone seemed to lose hope. There was nothing more the doctors could do.

'It was only when we gave up hoping that the Lord stepped in again and within three months I was pregnant. And thank goodness I was! The stress and strain, particularly this time round were almost unbearable. Medical tests, such as semen analysis and postcoital tests can really upset your sex life. So can the temperature charts, day in, day out waiting for the big moment. This is one area that doctors don't seem to be aware of. They are so keen to get you pregnant and put you down on their success list that they forget you are a human being with feelings. However desperate we were to be pregnant there were times when it was all too much for us to cope with.'

There is no doubt that the mental tensions can hinder the success of medical treatment and it is at times like these that the individual couple must withdraw, temporarily or permanently. We were forced to take 'time off', because our next appointment was in one year's time and looking back I can see that there was some value in this. At least it gave us the freedom to choose whether we used temperature charts or not and there was no pressure from repeat tests and waiting for results. It is not a bad idea to opt for a few months 'off duty' when the tensions get too great.

Some very dear friends, James and Emma spent four years on the medical merry-go-round and they are one of those couples for whom it is seemingly wasted. When they first sought help Emma was thirty and so the GP was prepared to move things along fairly fast. In addition, she worked as a medical secretary at the local hospital so she got red carpet treatment. Emma wrote, 'Being part of the establishment made things easier (except on one occasion when one of the students I knew well was on the clinic—he tactfully walked out). The staff were very helpful and because I could pop around the corner to see the technician when it was convenient, for example for postcoital tests, there was no waiting around.'

For many couples the long time waiting in clinics for tests to be carried out or to see doctors is one of the biggest areas of strain. Already under tension and maybe waiting in the antenatal room with a bevy of pregnant ladies, it can become almost claustrophobic. It can be nearly impossible to concentrate on reading a book and so every minute seems like an hour and resentment is added to the other frustrations.

Fortunately for James and Emma they had none of this, but then suddenly in the middle of examinations and investigations they had to move. This meant attending a different hospital in a new area.

'We had to wait six months for a transfer appointment, which didn't worry me at the time as I thought they were getting information from our previous hospital. However, when I actually went, the consultant whom I saw (and then didn't see again for two years), asked *me* what tests I'd had and what the results were. No information was ever asked for or received from our previous hospital.'

For the next two years Emma was seen by the registrar. After two postcoital tests, several hormone analyses, Fallopian tube x-ray, pituitary x-ray, semen analyses, and temperature charts, there just did not seem to be anything wrong. James said, 'On a physical plane we derived comfort from the knowledge that there was no irreversible problem to worry about. On the emotional and spiritual plane it was a very negative situation'.

Emma continued, 'Emotionally it was all very draining as nothing seemed to be wrong and so nothing seemed to be being done. The registrar obviously didn't know what to do or what to suggest, so he put me on a series of pills to 'boost things up'—but it didn't. I had Clomiphene 'on and off for about two years, at various rates and lengths, but all it did was to reduce my monthly cycle to about 16 days, which was a bit much!'

James went on to say, 'At this stage no advice was given and we had no idea what was going on. I do not feel that the staff have always been helpful. Sometimes there has been an off-handedness which I do not think has come up to professional standards.'

One of the GPs at their practice was amazed at the tests

that they had not had done (in my experience James and Emma were very thoroughly examined. Most couples do not get anywhere near as much attention and this would tend to indicate that infertility problems are given low priority in the medical world.) Emma pestered to see the consultant and when eventually she did, Artificial Insemination Husband (AIH)* was suggested. Nobody quite knows why.

James summed it up for me, 'The best hope is when the hospital gives up—now Emma's pregnant!'

Most couples will appreciate that sentiment. However helpful the medical staff, it is of necessity a long-winded process. The pressures of time and of money are such that appointments are few and far between and only a few selected tests are carried out for most couples. So far I have not met anyone who was dealt with in a systematic and logical sequence, who was kept sympathetically informed throughout. In most instances the tests carried out appear to be on the whim of the individual doctor and since there is seldom continuity of doctors this can be very random. A consultant that I saw much later on was staggered to discover that I was given a laparoscopy before any blood tests had been carried out and worse, that the results of Ian's semen analysis were not known at that time.

Infertility is a problem that is faced by 10-15% of the population, in some form or another. Charities such as CHILD[11] and the National Association for the Childless (NAC)[12] are fighting hard to remedy the lack of interest in the medical profession, but in the meantime there are many couples who are receiving inadequate treatment.

Whatever the medical outcome in the long-run, there are improvements which can be made today. There is no excuse for offhandedness and brusqueness, insensitivity and callousness. Every medical practitioner should be reminded that he or she is dealing with a human being with emotions and not just a case number.

A friend of mine, Veronica, had to go through the routine and was found to have two blocked fallopian tubes. After he told her the results, the doctor upset her by asking all manner of personal questions, including

'Have you had sexual intercourse with anyone other than your husband?' and 'Have you ever had V.D.?' explaining that blocked fallopian tubes could be the result of V.D. Veronica told me later, 'I was left feeling dirty. I felt guilty about something I hadn't done and somehow felt that he had cheapened my relationship with my husband. Whether he believed in my innocence or not, he certainly left me feeling very unclean.'

It was not until her next appointment, when Veronica saw the consultant, that she was told there were several causes of blocked fallopian tubes, from V.D. to a ruptured appendix or a severe urinary infection, but that it could also occur in women who had never experienced any known disease of the urinogenital tract.*

A recently published book by the Order of Christian Unity, includes this sentence at the beginning[13],

> 'Its application (i.e. IVF) to relieve infertility caused primarily by blockage of the fallopian tubes in the female, albeit that blockage has so often been caused by the patient's own prior fault, has nevertheless already brought untold happiness and relief to scores of childless couples . . . .'

Then later in the same book, in one of the papers given at the conference, we read,

> 'It happens that sometimes the Fallopian tubes are blocked, most often as a sequela of a sexually transmissable disease.'[14]

In neither case is the statement qualified nor handled with sensitivity and therefore could cause embarrassment and added hurt to a person who is already psychologically injured. I have one blocked fallopian tube, but it is my own prior fault and I strongly object to the underlying insinuations raised by such bald statements.

There are times when full information is needed, however hurtful the truth might be, and in some of these situations medical practitioners would be better understood if they used laymen's terms. Medical jargon can sound like a foreign language to the uninitiated and the use of initials, such as IVF, FSH, D&C, HCG*, has the sinister ring of a secret code used by the intelligentsia.

Doctors have a very difficult tight-rope to walk with regard to giving information. We want to know what is wrong with us, we want firm, reliable replies. When I asked the doctor what my chances of pregnancy were with one blocked fallopian tube, I wanted definite statistics, such as 50:50, but it is not that simple. Consequently many doctors return such nebulous replies that we feel they are not being truthful with us. We need to be ready to probe further and enquire whether the doctor is, in fact, withholding unpalatable information or whether he cannot be more specific because he doesn't know any more.

If we are truthful with ourselves, we often want to hear the things that please us and inadvertently encourage the doctor to raise false hopes. Later we are inclined to lay all the blame at his door. It is better in the long run to face the truth as soon as possible, and most couples will admit this.

Ray and Helen are a couple who were continually given false hopes. Theirs was not a problem of conception, because in fact Helen got pregnant very quickly. Theirs was a problem of genetic incompatability.* They have given birth to two hideously deformed babies who subsequently died and had two miscarriages that were quite probably also deformed.

After the first baby died, they were told that they had a fairly good chance of having a normal baby next time and that they should try again. A few months later Helen had her first miscarriage. She was taken to her local hospital for a D & C, but the staff did not check her medical history and so the foetus was not examined to see if it was also deformed. Nothing daunted they were advised to try again. The performance was repeated. Nobody knew whether this third foetus was also deformed.

This was very important, because if the foetus had been examined and found to be deformed, Helen could have been told that her chances of having a normal baby were being rapidly reduced. It is now thought that after her first baby she had a 1 in 20 chance of having a malformed baby by the time she had had two miscarriages, this was probably increased to a 1 in 3 chance.

However, Helen and Ray were not told any of this at the time, they were simply told to keep trying. Eventually Helen sustained a pregnancy but at the eighth month it was found to be badly deformed and so she was induced to give birth early. Nobody quite knows why the deformity was missed, because Helen underwent several scans as well as an amniocentesis. However, she believes that this was God's direct intervention because she feels she could never have countenanced an abortion.

Helen and Ray were at last given genetic counselling which at first they could not understand, because of its complexity, but eventually when they were sent to a specialist, it was explained in layman's terms. They began to understand that their chances of having a normal child were by now minimal, due to their genetic incompatibility. However, they were still given hope by the doctors and encouraged to keep trying.

The London hospital to which they had been referred, recommended that they should continue conceiving and that if a pregnancy was found to be deformed, the hospital would carry out an abortion, Helen said 'They forgot that we were human beings with feelings and emotions. They had never seen such bad genetic pairing and frankly they saw us as specimens that they could study. I see abortion as murder and so what they were suggesting was absolutely impossible for us, to say nothing of the emotional trauma we would have suffered. Still they told us there was a chance and so I was determined to go ahead and try once more, but on my own terms.'

However, it was at this point that the Lord intervened. Helen went to see her own GP who was a Christian and discussed the situation with him. Gently he suggested to her that she and Ray should think very carefully about their duty as Christians. He hinted that maybe it was God's plan that they should not have children of their own. He then, wisely, advised her to go away and convalesce. Helen went to her mother-in-law's home and whilst there she was seen by an ex-missionary doctor.

This man was absolutely forthright and told her that they should have no more children. He reminded her that they were themselves children of the Lord and as such they should be ready to submit to His will. He told her to think carefully about whether it was right to run the risk of bringing another deformed baby into the world. He encouraged her not to have any false hopes and assured her that God would give them the grace to accept His will.

Ray and Helen were devastated and yet they knew that this man was right. Together after much prayer and heart-searching they made the decision not to try again and with that decision came peace. Today they have two beautiful adopted children, and can truly rejoice in what the Lord has done for them.

False hopes such as these and mistakes such as the foetus that were not examined are unnecessary and require no major changes in the system to be put right. Money could be saved by doing tests in the right order, semen analyses are easier and cheaper to do than postcoital tests or laparoscopys. Unnecessary tests could be avoided.

Nevertheless it is now estimated that about 50 per cent of the couples who attend hospital for treatment can be helped in one way or another and this is very encouraging. The medical profession do have a lot to offer and not least is the feeling that something positive is being done.

The question is not so much whether one should seek medical help, but how long one should persevere with it. The emotional and spiritual strain, plus the strain that it can put on a marriage, is very great and each couple must decide for themselves when they have had enough and not be ashamed to admit it.

Practical hints on surviving the medical merry-go-round

1 Don't get too anxious about treatment at hospitals—so far as they are concerned we are sausages in a machine. Accept that before you go and don't expect too much.
2 For most couples the outcome is positive, so don't give up hope—try to give up worrying instead!

3 If you do not feel that you are getting adequate help ask to see the consultant—and keep pestering.
4 If you don't understand the things you are being told ask them to explain in laymen's terms. If you are not being told anything start asking questions!
5 If you are asked to take tests or treatment that you are not happy about don't be afraid to ask for time to think about it. If you want to get off the roundabout for a while, say so. It's your body, your marriage, your right.
6 Try to keep a sense of humour. It can be very traumatic and many of the questions and tests are very personal. Try to laugh about it.
7 When attending appointments go together as a couple if you can. Often both are needed, but even if only the woman is required she may well benefit from her husband's support, during or after the event.
8 Read 'Why US?' by Dr Andrew Stanway[2]. This is an excellent book setting out medical procedure, explaining medical terminology and advising you on what to expect and look out for.
9 Before you go too far discuss together and if necessary with your pastor or some other sympathetic and respected Christian, the ethics of the various medical treatments. Be positive about what you believe and how far you are willing to go and stand by it.

5. Interrogation: Questions

Parents In A Quandary

This child needs a good home
Security
Love
This child needs real parents
Mummy
Daddy

This child has a need

We need a family
Son
Daughter
We need someone to love
Hold
Cherish

We need a child

Child meet my need
We'll meet your need

I must remember this
I must hold on to this,
In the days of waiting,
waiting,
waiting.

I am sick of all the questions
How?
When?
Where?
Why?
Do you?
Could you?
Would you?
Should you?

I don't know any more.
At first we saw so clearly
Now we are surrounded by dense fog.

I don't know what I would do
If a child emptied jam on the carpet
        threw a temper tantrum in church
        deliberately cut up my curtains
Give me that child
Mine
To love
And I will tell you how I will react.

Lord, give me patience
            tact
            foresight.

Child, I will meet your need—in time.

Some months previously it had been suggested to us that if we were really anxious to have a family we should consider a proxy family. To be truthful, at first, like many other women, I was not at all keen on the idea. I was not prepared to give up hope that we would have children of our own and for some reason I felt that to begin fostering or adopting would be to betray my hope.

Ian thought that was ridiculous and urged me to think out my reasons, to talk about them and to pray about them. Maybe it was ridiculous but that was the way I felt. Now I find that I am not alone. Sue told me that 'I would never have considered adopting, not for one moment. I don't think adoption is for everyone and it certainly wasn't for me.' She gave no reasons, it was just a 'gut reaction'.

Emma was rather more honest. She said, 'For us the problem has always been infertility, not childlessness. We never seriously considered the possibility that we might not have children and so we never seriously considered adoption. But anyway, my initial feeling was that I didn't want another woman's unwanted child. I guess if we had really been brought to the crunch we would have considered a third world adoption or a half-caste.'

Deep down inside many of us feel the same way as Emma in the first instance. People who advise adoption or fostering as one of the primary solutions to childlessness do not take into account the desires of the couple. Primarily a married couple seek to fulfil one of the purposes of marriage:

> 'It was ordained for the increase of mankind, and that children might be brought up in the fear and nurture of the Lord.'[1]

So the initial desire is to have a child of your own, your own flesh and blood. Once you have a child of your own, you can more compassionately consider adoption from the point of view of the needs and desires of the child. Once you have been told that there is no hope you can also admit that you want a family and that here is a means to an end.

That all sounds very clinical and callous, but it is in fact a natural feeling and not one to be ashamed of. Very few couples can consider the question less subjectively and for them adoption is as natural as giving birth and so is right, regardless of whether they ever have children of their own.

It was said to us that there were so many unwanted children in the world that we should take advantage of our childlessness to offer 'a good Christian home' to one of these deprived children. Who can deny that there are many unhappy, unwanted, underprivileged children? In Britain alone there are said to be some 20,000 'hard-to-place' children (that is coloured, handicapped or several siblings) all desperately needing loving homes. As Christians we all have a responsibility to these children, not just those suffering from infertility.

Before an infertile couple can consider fostering or adoption seriously, they must first be allowed to grieve for the child they cannot have. They must be surrounded by love, care, sympathy and understanding until they personally are ready.

It has been said that 'all children come as gifts of God to parents and whether they are delivered by one route or another, they are no less our very own.'[15] To this we all come, but only after healing by the Holy Spirit of our own hurt and broken spirits.

So I worked through my emotions, my fears, my hesitancy. I began to wonder whether, in fact, we had been allowed to go through our experiences in order that we would consider fostering or adoption. I began to realize that I was not betraying my hope, that I could still continue trying for a family of my own, that I could still seek medical help, that this was not an end but merely another step.

I began to see that I could use this time constructively for the Lord and that instead of stifling my maternal instincts I would be better to put them to good use. Already I had gone back into creche work at my church, with this in mind and I had just taken on a new post in a children's hospital. This would be just another step in the same direction.

The decision was finally made when I rang the social services to make preliminary enquiries and was told that the whole process could take two years; one year to be approved and then a year before a child was placed with us. It seemed right to go ahead and continue testing the Lord as we went.

We were very fortunate that the social services responded so positively. Many couples have told me that they are less than encouraging to couples who have no children. The reason appears to be that there are very few white, healthy babies available and this is what the childless couple usually want. In 1979, a quarter of a million couples queued for some 5000 babies.[4] Most of the babies and children readily available for adoption are mentally or physically handicapped or coloured, or in groups of siblings or are a mixture of these.

We did not try other adoption societies at this stage. In retrospect I think this was probably because we were only putting out feelers, testing God in a way. Had we been utterly convinced that God intended us to adopt we would probably have written to some of the Christian societies. Today most of these societies have closed their books and so the outlook is not very hopeful.

In the first instance a man and a woman from the social services came to visit us in our own home. They spent the time explaining terminology, discussing the procedure, timing and giving us some case histories. They showed us an album full of children mostly coloured, siblings or hard-to-place, and then asked us if we still wanted to go ahead. They recommended that we went for long-term fostering with a view to adoption, rather than short-term fostering or straightforward adoption.

Short-term fostering is when a child, of any age from babyhood up to a maximum of eighteen, is placed with a family for an unknown period of time. This can be anything from a day to six months and can be used for a variety of reasons. For example, at that time there were three siblings who had to be taken in for fostering because the mother was in hospital and the father could not cope. There was also a newly born baby who would probably be up for adoption but the mother kept changing her mind.

At first this appealed strongly to me, because I felt that it was something I could get involved with but without the long-term commitment. If I should fall pregnant then we would be able to request that no more children be sent to us. However, the social worker was strongly against this, for two main reasons. Firstly, she felt that as we had no children of our own I would get too attached and be unwilling to surrender a child, and secondly she obviously felt we had no experience of parenting and would therefore only be of limited value in this field.

Long-term fostering is where a child is placed with a family for at least six months and usually for some years.

Often these are children who will eventually be adopted, but for whom there is a legal battle going on, or some other complication. Legally if the child remains with the foster family for a consecutive period of five years the foster family can go to court and request legal adoption.

In this instance the couple decide what kind of child they are willing to take. The social services then find a suitable child and a period of visiting and adjustment is undertaken. If both parents and child are happy then the placement is made. In general, these are children who are 'hard-to-place'. They may be of another race, of mixed parenthood, they may be older white children who have often been in several short-stay foster homes, or they may have physical or mental problems.

Adoption is where a child is immediately available for legal adoption and the procedure is much the same as for long-term fostering. In general, those who seek adoption are wanting babies and as there is quite a long waiting list for white, healthy babies many couples are encouraged to foster.

We finally agreed to apply for 'long-term fostering with a view to adoption' and so the screening began. This is very taxing for there is no such thing as privacy and we soon found every corner of our lives being vetted. All our thoughts, feelings, hopes, fears, motives were dragged out, exposed, dissected and psycho-analysed. If all parents-to-be had to undergo the same sort of cross-questioning there would be a rapid fall in the birth rate.

The social worker visited us once a fortnight and we soon discovered that we were his first 'case'. Consequently he was absolutely meticulous with us, asking every question in detail, taking copious notes and never letting the smallest thing go. We soon felt that social workers have no sense of humour and we began to think that their aim was to put you off.

Increasingly we were made to feel that they were doing us a great favour by screening us and that if ever we were approved it would be a great condescension on their part and we would be indebted to them for whatever child we were offered. Their attitude gave the impression that there were hundreds of desperate couples waiting to be given a child and I often wondered why there were always adverts in the local paper.

At this point we sought reassurance about what we were doing and it was suggested that we might talk to other foster or adoptive parents. The social services hold regular parents meetings so that people can share their experiences together for mutual encouragement and support. However, there was not one scheduled for some time so our social worker arranged for us to visit the home of a couple who had done short-term fostering for some years and were now taking a three-year-old boy for adoption.

We were told in advance that Gary had been left by his parents whilst a baby and had woken up to find himself looking into the face of a stranger. He was short-term fostered while the social services sought to have him taken into permanent care. For the three short years of Gary's life, he had been shunted from foster home to foster home. Now he was totally introverted—he could not or would not speak, he was naughty in the extreme and very difficult to handle. At last he was up for adoption.

Ann and Simon, his adoptive parents-to-be, made us feel instantly at home and were delighted to share with us from their experience. They had decided that they would take a child for adoption and because of their vast experience of fostering they were asked to take Gary. At first, Ann and Simon were rather hesitant but finally they agreed to meet him. Ann told us that she 'fell for him' immediately and knew that however hard it was and however long it took she would have Gary. They started by visiting the little boy once a week. Then when Gary began to recognise them, Ann was allowed to take him out for an hour, then half a day, then a whole day and finally for a week-end. The visits became more frequent as Gary responded and accepted them, until Ann was seeing him almost daily.

From the start Gary had been a little demon, but as he came to accept Ann, be began to feel more secure and so his bad behaviour improved slightly. Now they had him home for a trial period of a whole week.

I watched as Gary careered around the small living

room, leaping on and off the seats, hurling toys, clambering onto Simon's lap and sliding off again almost before he had got up. Suddenly, he stopped by the table, picked up the sugar basin and emptied it right in the middle of the floor. I waited with held breath. Nothing happened. There was no retribution, Ann just quietly got to her feet, fetched a brush and dustpan and cleared up. Gary giggled loudly and jumped from one foot to the other.

To be honest I was horrified. How could they both be so calm? Was this his normal behaviour? Then an interesting thing happened.

Just as Ann sat down again this noisy little boy began to gabble. Nothing was intelligible to me, but it was obvious that these sounds were different from the others, he was trying to communicate. Ann and Simon seemed to understand and Ann put out her arms to Gary. Delighted he ran across the room and climbed onto her lap, where he curled up like a puppy dog. It seemed that after all these months Gary really was trying to talk. It was the gibberish of a fifteen-month-old, but much more exciting. He was disciplined for serious naughtiness, but patience with the small mischiefs and a constant unswerving love was winning through to this mixed-up lad.

By the time we left, my mind was in turmoil. I knew that I wasn't ready for a Gary and yet Ann and Simon's enthusiasm and encouragement had excited me. We talked long and late that night and finally concluded that natural parents could face similar problems. We were horrified by the enormity of the task and yet conversely we were even more determined to continue the screening.

What we had been through with the medical profession was nothing compared to the vetting by the social services. We were asked intimate questions that bore little or no relevance to fostering a child. I failed to see that the intimacies of our sex life would affect our ability to be good parents. I did not understand why the form required that we give the names and addresses of all the members of our family and their qualifications and job status. I could not quite comprehend why they filled in another form which was thirty-six pages long.

Of course they needed a medical reference and we had to have another medical examination. I could accept that they had to check with the police that we had no criminal record, but we also had to have two character references, from people who had known us well for two years. Do I sound bitter? Well, I guess I was. It was very gruelling at a time when we were already vulnerable.

Our lives were becoming an open book and at times we both wondered whether to stop the procedure. I remember that after the evening discussing our private lives, my husband shut the front door after the social worker and let out a blood curdling yell. It took more than half an hour to calm him down and all my powers of persuasion to get him to the next meeting! We tried approaching one or two private adoption agencies at this point but they all replied that their books were closed.

We persevered. From the very beginning we had been totally honest about our love of the Lord and our involvement with a church. At first the social worker had 'reassured' us that the committee 'usually looked kindly' on Christians. However, as the time passed we began to realize that he was becoming increasingly obsessed with our commitment.

To be truthful I wondered whether he was actually searching for the truth and so kept asking detailed questions about our beliefs. We had nothing to be ashamed of and answered him openly on all fronts. However, as time passed we realized that he was actually worried stiff about our commitment. Almost every meeting he would bring the conversation round to our beliefs and repeatedly asked whether we would expect a child to go to church with us. He was obviously worried about 'indoctrination'.

After six months he decided he was ready to present his 'case' to the board. We were told the date of the meeting and that he would ring us the following day. He did ring us, to say that the second social worker, who had only visited us twice had gone on holiday without submitting our report, so our case had not been heard. We would have to wait another month.

This did not worry us too much. Things were happening

in other parts of our lives which made us willing to wait for the Lord's time. The month was soon over and the social worker rang. Please could he come and see us to discuss the outcome—we had not been turned down, but...

It transpired that there were three points the committee wanted clarified.

1 The social worker had not seen our marriage certificate, had we got one?
2 Ian had once said he didn't see why the law should dictate the age at which a child should be told he was adopted. Did this mean he would not tell the child, because that was illegal?
3 They were worried about our church involvement.

I was speechless, which was fortunate. Ian, however, was quick to reply with heavy sarcasm. 1. No, we were not married. 2. Why should he? 3. What did they want to know because we would be happy to discuss our faith at length.

Our social worker came and we spent the whole evening discussing our faith, our church, our commitment, our attitudes towards upbringing and so on. Ground we had covered again and again. Exhausted he went away to write his supplementary report. Later we discovered that the committee included several church members and clergymen, so why the inquisition? We still do not know the answer, but our case was approved with no trouble the next time. We were completely drained, but we were approved foster parents. Now all we had to do was wait for a child.

Tom and Sarah are going through the mill at the moment. Nothing has changed during the last four years. They describe it as a humiliating experience and one that they would not put up with if it were not for the end in view. They do not know whether they will be accepted, but they have an interesting problem.

Tom and Sarah live in a small town, in beautiful English countryside. Their's is not a cosmopolitan area, and to date there are no coloured people. They have been told by their social worker that many of the available children are coloured or half-caste. What are they to do? They say,

'We are not colour prejudiced and if we lived in an area

with a mixed population we would not hesitate. But how can we adopt an Asian or West Indian child? He or she would be the only one at school, the only one in the neighbourhood, is that really fair?

We have had to say that we will only take a white child and we have been told that this probably means a physically or mentally handicapped child. We have no children of our own, we have never been parents. We don't know how to bring up a normal healthy child, so will we be able to cope with a handicapped one?'

Sarah went on to say that she had found the whole procedure very gruelling. 'The visitors we have had have always been kind and considerate, but I got a bit impatient with the sort of questions we were asked and I found the forms we had to fill in verging on the impossible! One of the things I found the hardest to answer was why I wanted to adopt children, in fact why I wanted children. I don't see why the fact that you are seeking to adopt a child means that you want him for any different reason than you would want a natural child.'

I do not entirely agree with Sarah. Personally I wanted my own child as a fulfilment of my God-given purpose. I wanted the experience, thrill and joy of pregnancy. I wanted to use my female body for one of the purposes for which it was created. I wanted Ian's child because I love him, he is my husband and only he could fulfil these bodily needs and desires. But then when we did not conceive new reasons began to surface.

I didn't like being different. I wanted to be like all my friends. I didn't like the thought that we couldn't do what everyone else seemed to be experts at—that is making a baby. I didn't like the thought that we would always be alone, I wanted the joy of a family. I didn't want to be a career woman, a dietician—even a District Dietician. I wanted to be a wife and mother, I wanted to make a home. All these desires could be fulfilled by an adopted or fostered child and in addition I could use our situation for the benefit of an unloved and unwanted child. The previous reasons for wanting a child could not be fulfilled by adoption.

Sarah also reminded me of one other thing and that is

the fact that the adoption panel accepts or rejects a couple and that their decision is final. However, from our own experience the panel may request further information before making a negative decision and so this can lead to final acceptance. Nevertheless once a couple are actually rejected, no appeal is allowed and no reasons for the decision are given. This can be devastating.

It is fair to say, however, that most interviewers learn to read a couple accurately and where there is serious doubt, then the interviewer will usually try to stop the couple proceeding. They cannot refuse outright to present your case, but you can be sure that if you have to hold a gun at their head to get them to agree to put you before the panel then your case is already lost! If you survive the interviews and your case is taken before the panel by an enthusiastic interviewer then it is probable that you will be accepted.

Alison and Mark had a long wait and extra medicals before they were finally accepted. They decided to adopt when they were told that there was no hope of their being able to conceive a child. Alison wrote to forty different societies, but only one had its books open at the time. The social services had 'such a negative attitude' that it put them off completely and so they opted to go through this one agency.

Alison and Mark were prepared for a long wait and so were taken completely by surprise when they received a letter inviting them to a group meeting. Alison said, 'The social services had so put us off that we were beginning to feel very negative and to wonder whether this really was the right thing for us. However, we felt that we ought to attend the meeting and we are so glad we did. We both came out with all our original enthusiasm.'

They had the usual interviews and forms to fill in, although these were apparently much shorter and dealt with in a much more sympathetic manner. Then they suffered a set-back. Due to Mark's illness they were asked to have a special medical examination by the society's doctor. The outcome of this was that they were asked to wait two years, to be sure that Mark's illness had been contained.

This was a very desolate time. They had patiently accepted all the questioning, feeling that every question was a step nearer having the family they longed for. Now they were filled with a feeling of helplessness and horror at the long wait ahead of them. They had also been told that even if they were accepted at the end of the two years, they would probably have to wait another six months or more until a baby was found for them.

However, they soon saw God's hand at work, because Mark suddenly became seriously ill and Alison found that all her time and energy was spent on him. 'In a funny sort of way my maternal instincts were fulfilled by caring for him. There was no room for other thoughts.'

Mark recovered and then they had another surprise letter, inviting Mark to come for his final medical. It was only eighteen months. There was no hitch and they were accepted and settled back for the final lap. It was to be a mere six weeks before Alison received a phone call from her social worker to ask if they could take month-old twin boys in four days time. Alison was filled with horror and a sense of inadequacy and nearly refused them in her fright.

However, they brought the boys home and then the sense of helplessness really did envelope her. 'I had become very hesitant about picking up other people's children and had particular problems with babies. It was a reflex action to prevent myself getting hurt. Now I was presented with two tiny babies and I really had to steel myself to pick them up.

For three weeks it was sheer murder. When one stopped crying the other started. There was always a nappy to be changed or a bottle to be made up. I was so tired and I wasn't getting a full night's sleep. I didn't feel that I loved them as I should and I began to get more and more het up. Finally I decided I just couldn't cope, that we had made a mistake, that I would never be a mother.

Fortunately we had a Christian doctor who called to see me. He gave me two sleeping tablets and told Mark and Grandma to take over. I slept and slept and when I woke up everything was different. I am now totally committed to my sons and love them deeply. I am determined to give them the best I have to give, to be utterly consistent in my dealings with them and my discipline. They are very, very special and have brought release for us both.'

Many infertile couples, who finally have a family by whatever means feel this extra commitment towards the child. Ray and Helen are just the same. After their second baby died and they were counselled not to have any more they decided to go forward for adoption.

They also wrote to a large number of adoption societies and finally found one that was just opening its books again after two years of closure. They were among the twelve couples selected from 40,000 applicants. They had three interviews along with the usual references and medicals, but they found that the whole procedure was handled in a friendly, homely manner and sensitive areas were dealt with gently and speedily.

The first interview was in February and they were accepted in July, when there was still a nine-month waiting list. However, four months later a baby girl was placed with them and Helen describes the timing as perfect. Like Alison she could not face newborn babies and found that their crying could send her into utter despair. However, as she learnt to love and care for her new daughter healing came. Now they have an adopted son too and Helen is completely healed, even though she knows that she can never have her own child.

It is a fact that adoption can be the very best means of healing. Alison knows that God chose the twins especially for them and set them aside as a couple to be their parents. It is a real calling for her and in it she is completely contented.

Despite the long period of assessment, the probing questions the inevitable time lag, adoption and fostering are positive solutions. They should not be entered into lightly and the couple should have support from their families and their spiritual counsellor throughout. Adoption and fostering are Biblical principles, but this does not mean that they are right for all couples. Those who are called to this vocation, will be greatly blessed, but those who are not called should not be ashamed to say so and should not be pressurized by society or other Christians.

Practical hints about adoption and fostering

1 Write to as many societies as you can find, but don't be disappointed if most of them have closed their books. You only need one opening. There is no doubt that Christian or private societies are much more considerate and understanding in their handling of the questions. Conversely, they often have less children available.

2 If you are uncertain about whether this is right for you ask if there is a group meeting of foster/adoptive parents that you can attend, or whether there are foster parents who will talk to you. This is most helpful as it gives you the chance to ask questions and to see a working relationship.

3 The questions will be intimate and may seem offensive. Keep a keen sense of humour, remember that each question brings you a step nearer and don't be afraid to parry a question. Some social workers get carried away with their role and it may be that there are some situations where you would be better to answer with a question of your own.

4 You will have to have two referees who know you well. Be sure they understand why you are seeking to adopt/foster.

5 When you are offered a child spend as much time as possible with him/her. If it is a child with problems this is even more important.

6 Don't be afraid to say no. It is better to admit your hesitation than to take the child and have to admit defeat after six months or a year.

7 Remember, when the time comes you will feel totally inadequate, helpless and maybe even have a sense of horror at the enormity of the task. This is all quite natural and providing you are not being persuaded to take a child against your will, you will soon find that your natural instincts come to the fore and you will be able to love the child.

8 Call in the 'emergency squad'. If this is your first child

you will be exhausted, emotionally, physically and even spiritually. Make sure Grandma, a neighbour or friend is at the ready to give you a break. Sleep is a marvellous healer.

6. Devastation: Spiritual Depression

Complaint To My Father

I can't love you, Lord.
Not right now.
I am too angry,
too hurt,
too confused.

Why, Lord?
Why have you, a God of Love,
allowed this to happen to me?

Why am I denied this blessing?
Your blessing,
You ordained marriage, for procreation,
You are the giver,
why withhold the gift?

I can't understand,
I am floundering,
in a theological morass
sinking
into the mud
of misbelief.

Is it me?
Is it him?

Can we change your mind?
Is it right?
Is it sin?
Can you heal our mind?

Help me,
I cannot hold on much longer,
Put your arms beneath me
lest I fall
and am broken
irrepairably.

Don't let go
please
Don't let go
I'll be alright
in time

Tomorrow
I will have faith
Tomorrow
Hold me
Til then

Let me cry
in your arms
safe
until I can love you
again.

Four months after we first began the adoption procedure, I was once more pregnant and it seemed that God was answering our prayer. By now I was longing more than ever that we could have our own child and a large part of the reason was that I was keen to tell the social worker to move on! We were also going through a rather dry spiritual patch, carrying out a superficial religiosity, while our hearts were cold.

It is always difficult to remember that we are whole people and that when we are mentally and physically depressed, we can easily become spiritually depressed. We had lost sight of this home truth and were beginning to feel very isolated. Our prayers became endless repititions of the same request, 'Please Lord give us a baby'. We never doubted that he was God, but we did doubt his love. Our quiet time had dwindled to that one priority prayer. We were so wrapped up in our need that we could hardly spare the time to pray for anyone else.

We had come to the conclusion that God was not going to give us our heart's desire just for the asking. We were going to have to badger Him to change His mind. Together we read the story of the widow in Luke 18. 3 - 7:

> 'And there was a widow in that town who kept coming to him with the plea, "Grant me justice against my adversary."
> For some time he (the Judge) refused. But finally he said to himself, 'even though I don't fear God or care about men, yet because this widow keeps bothering me, I will see that she gets justice, so that she won't eventually wear me out with her coming!"
> And the Lord said, "Listen to what the unjust judge says, and will not God bring about justice for his chosen ones, who cry out to him day and night? Will he keep putting them off? I tell you, he will see that they get justice and quickly." ' (NIV)

And again we read in Luke 11 5 - 10:

> 'Then he said to them, "Suppose one of you has a friend and he goes to him at midnight and says, "Friend lend me three loaves of bread, because a friend of mine on a journey has come to me, and I have nothing to set before him.
> Then the one inside answers, "Don't bother me. The door is already locked, and my children are with me in bed. I can't get up and give you anything." I tell you though he will not get up and give him the bread because he is his friend, yet because of the man's persistence he will get up and give him as much as he needs."

So I say to you: ask and it will be given you . . . .
For everyone who asks receives . . . ' (NIV)

So we prayed endlessly, not knowing why we were being kept waiting, not understanding the ways of the Lord and yet determined to wear down His resistance!

At last, it seemed that our prayers were answered and our perseverance rewarded. But then at seven weeks I began to miscarry. This time I went straight to my bed and the GP agreed to total bed-rest, until she could visit in a couple of days. We alerted the family to pray and searched the scriptures again and again.

We read the story of the Shunamite woman (2 Kings 4. 8-37). She was another of the barren women mentioned and had regularly given hospitality to Elisha. He had wanted to do something for her and his servant told him that she had no child.

'Elisha said (to her), "About this time next year, you will hold a son in your arms."
"No, my lord," she objected. "Don't mislead your servant, O man of God! . . . . Don't raise my hopes." '
(2 Kings 4. 16 and 28b NIV)

We cried the same thing to the Lord. We begged Him not to let us lose this child. Why raise our hopes if it was to end the same way? I wept silently as I lay and Ian turned to a passage of encouragement, Luke 11. 11-13:

'Which of you fathers, if your son asks for a fish, will give him a snake instead? Or if he asks for an egg, will give him a scorpion? If you then, though you are evil, know how to give good gifts to your children how much more will your father in heaven, give the Holy Spirit to those who ask him!' (NIV)

We hoped, but again we lost the baby. Our weak faith crumbled like the flakiest pastry, as we simply could not understand why God had allowed this to happen to us.

> 'For my thoughts are not your thoughts neither are your ways my ways, declares the Lord. As the heavens are higher than the earth so are my ways higher than your ways and my thoughts than your thoughts. . . . . my word that goes out from my mouth: It will not return to me empty, but will accomplish what I desire and achieve the purpose for which I sent it you will go out in joy and be led forth in peace.'
> (Isaiah 55. 8 - 12 NIV)

If only we could have taken that promise for ourselves, but we were too disappointed, our faith too weak. It was to be another six months before we could truly take this word to our hearts.

Our families surrounded us by love and support. Many tried to encourage us and we were told that there was a purpose in all this. That God was refining us, for service and that because of this we would one day be able to help others. Was Hannah told the same thing? Did it comfort her to think this? I doubt it, for although what she suffered helped me, over 2000 years later, I cannot perceive that had she known it would have soothed her pain. Neither did it soothe mine. Now, nearly four years later I can see the hand of God, I know His goodness, but then I was too depressed to think positively.

We shunned the help we were offered, because none had trodden our road. Those who came to comfort had children of their own. How could they understand the depth of our feelings?

Why was God denying us this simple request? We were not asking for anything abnormal or extravagant. A loving God, who is Himself a father, would surely not withhold this precious gift? I blamed God for what we were suffering and even hated Him. Then I felt guilty for this unprecedented feeling. Immediately I became obsessed with my sinfulness and this was a great stumbling block. In our distress, we withdrew into our shells, communicating only on a superificial level with those around us, denying the hurt. Our only conversations with the Lord were ones of anger and recriminations. We caused him a lot of sadness.

However much we may look back and wish that our faith had been stronger, what we went through was normal. We were physically and emotionally depressed and it was inevitable that we should also become spiritually depressed.

Sue and John are in the ministry and yet they too went through a spiritual black patch. John always believed that God was going to answer their prayers in the end, but he did wonder what He was trying to achieve in the interim. Sue had deeper problems, with which her husband could not help her. She had to see it through.

'I got to the stage where I simply couldn't be bothered with God. In my readings of the scriptures I found that children were a blessing from the Lord;

> "Sons are a heritage from the Lord,
> children a reward from Him . . . .
> Blessed is the man
> whose quiver is full of them." (Psalm 127.
> 3 & 5 NIV)

Did this mean that barrenness was a curse? What sin had I or we committed, how had we angered God? Quiet times were a real struggle and the only thing I could think of was to pray for a baby.'

Sue had no spiritual counselling; as the minister's wife, to whom could she go? During her really black patches, her husband would pray with her, hour after hour until she was given some measure of peace. When she finally got pregnant and was anxious about the outcome she clung to the passage in Isaiah 66. 9:

> 'Do I bring to the moment of birth and not give delivery?
> says the Lord
> Do I close up the womb when I bring to delivery?
> says your God' (NIV)

Just before each of their babies was born she was given a specific word, which was a reminder to hang on to the

Lord however slender the thread that binds you at that time:

'No longer will Jacob be ashamed . . . .
When they see among them their children,
the work of my hands
they will keep my name holy;
they will acknowledge the holiness of the Holy
    One of Jacob
and will stand in awe of the God of Israel.'
(Isaiah 29. 22 NIV)

When I asked James and Emma how they had coped spiritually during their four and a half year wait, James, another minister replied,
'Problems? ME? No! A minister isn't allowed problems—is he? I could pray about it and occasionally talk to a friend, but I don't know what else I could have done. I suppose, I could have gone to a colleague, but then I am caught up in the myth that people have about the problemless minister.'

James did have times of struggling with his faith and of questioning the Lord. 'There was one question I wanted God to answer. In the marriage service, one of the preamble comments is that marriage is given for the birth and nurture of children. He had called us into marriage—so why withhold this gift? He knows best and I didn't get a very clear answer, or maybe I was deaf to it. Sometimes faith has been almost academic, instead of from the heart, I have always believed that God really does know best, but in prayer it is tempting to ask him to be a rubber stamp!'

Ian and I had often felt guilty about our doubting, anger, lack of faith and so on. James said, 'I didn't feel guilty. I have often told others and myself to be absolutely one hundred percent honest with God. He made me what I am, He gave me my feelings. If He made me this way, why should I be guilty? The main thing is to keep talking to God, tell Him openly exactly what you are feeling and why. Never lose touch.'

Every couple who have spoken to me, or written to me about this subject have admitted to times of deep spiritual depression. Most couples go through the stage of asking God, Why? Why me, Lord? Why allow it at all? Many go on from there to ask, Why won't God bless us? What have we done wrong?

Helen faced this question after the death of her first child. She sought the answer in Genesis 3, where she was reminded that man had sinned and that therefore we live in a fallen world. We reap what we have sown. God allows this to happen, but He will give us the grace to cope with it. She said,

'I knew the answer in my head but my heart cried out against it. No logical answer can ever relieve the pain in your heart, only God can heal there.'

During Helen's fourth pregnancy (she was still childless), she threatened to miscarry repeatedly throughout the first trimester and was confined to bed for several weeks. She and Ray prayed twice daily that God would make them willing to give this baby up to Him, if that was what He wanted. In the end it was what He wanted.

At eight months they were told that this baby was also hideously deformed and advised to have an induction. For one week they both walked around in a complete dream, knowing that this was God's will and yet not knowing how to accept it. For Ray this was worse than all the others, because he knew what Helen was going to go through and he longed that he might now carry her burden. There was only God left.

On the morning of the induction Helen and Ray were sleeping late. Suddenly Helen awoke to the sound of someone calling her name. She thought it was Ray. Helen did not want to wake up to this day. She was frightened of what she was going to have to go through, of a labour which was to be for nothing. She lay still, but again she heard her name being called, 'Helen, Helen!' Reluctantly she opened her eyes and became aware of an intense white light filling the room. She sat up, as though to see better and then the voice spoke again,

> 'Fear not, for I have redeemed you;
> I have called you by name, you are mine.

When you pass through the waters I will be with you; and through the rivers, they shall not overwhelm you; when you walk through fire you shall not be burned, and the flame shall not consume you. For I am the Lord your God, the Holy One of Israel, your Saviour.'

As Helen watched, the white light faded and the room came back, as though into focus. She woke Ray to tell him what had happened and although he himself had not heard the voice, he was comforted by Helen's peace. Throughout the day Helen was aware of God's presence as though he walked at her side, His arms about her. She was confident in the power of God and as she went into the anaesthetic there was no blackness only a white light and a voice which said, 'Underneath are the everlasting arms' and then again she heard the same words that she had heard that morning, the words from Isaiah 43. 1 - 3.

When Helen awoke it was to the feeling that she was still being cradled and she was able to hold on to the knowledge that God loved her and had kept her close.

Helen was to remember this in the weeks ahead, for her time of deepest trouble was still to come. She was soon advised by her Christian doctors not to have any more children. The crunch had come. Was she willing to submit totally to God? This was a time of utter desolation and they had two clear choices; to fall or to cling on to God. They chose to cling tightly. At night, when she was swamped by misery and depression she would cry out, calling on the name of the Lord and she would feel again the everlasting arms cradling her, feel again the warmth and the love bringing back security.

Helen was given two books to read. One was the story of Joni Eareckson,[16] the other was the story of Corrie Ten Boom,[17]. She was dismayed that the main theme running through both stories was to 'rejoice at all times and in all things give thanks to the Lord.' How, she cried could she rejoice and give thanks? She could praise God in an abstract way, but surely no-one would expect her to thank God for her deformed babies?

Then she read how Corrie had argued with her sister.

She would thank God for anything, everything, but she would not thank Him for the fleas. But it was the fleas which kept the guards away and gave the sisters greater freedom to witness. Helen and Ray got the message and from then on, when times were low they would say 'Thank you for the fleas.'

Now she can thank God from her heart. She knows that her babies are in heaven and healed and that her Father has them close to Himself. 'I know that one day I shall see them and they will be beautiful. This has made me realize that God has forged an unbreakable link between us and Himself and so now we are totally dependent on Him. This was God's only way to get us so close and dependent on Him. I feel privileged and so cherished.' Helen gives all the glory to God.

It is only in retrospect that most of us can acknowledge that God does know best, that He is right and to Him be the glory. At the time we can only hang on. Alison and Mark hung on throughout all the long wait for the adoption to be completed and throughout the fears engendered by Mark's illness.

Despite the fact that they were told fairly early on that Mark could never have children, they still believed that God had planned a child for them. They held on to this conviction and they knew that they must keep their faith, but at times they were very vulnerable. At these times they sought spiritual counsel and were strengthened by it. Most couples do not get adequate spiritual counselling. Their minister told me that on no account would he preach on such a subject from the pulpit. 'The pulpit is for the wider principles of the gospel. I will preach on marriage, but I will not preach on infertility, for this is an abnormal situation, and the problem of a few. However, I strongly believe that we have a responsibility to help in cases such as these, and I believe that the place to do this is in the fellowship groups, where there is a family atmosphere, or on a one to one personal counselling basis.'

Alison and Mark were generally supported by this man, who has a large family and yet had the ability to understand and feel their problems. He could weep with those who weep. This is some of the advice he gave, 'You will always feel inadequate or feel the lack of fulfilment with the burden of other people's comments. This can lead to inner resentment and this resentment must be dealt with. Now you have three choices of how you are going to deal with this.

Firstly you may pour it out to others. This will be seen in your attitudes and your reactions and the way you deal with people.

Secondly, you may keep it to yourself, so that it festers inside you, until finally you cannot respond to the love of God. Your hearts will be cold and you will be hardened against the Lord.

Thirdly, you can pour out to God your complaint, like the psalmist did. We have a Father. An atheist has no one to complain to, but we have a Father to complain to. When a child comes in tears and cries 'Why Mummy?', what do you do? You put your arms about the child and give him a big hug. Maybe it is too difficult to explain why, but you can comfort. So, in humility, broken-hearted you can go to the Father. Like the psalmist in Psalm 13, we can come crying and then God meets us half way and we can rejoice, He may not remove the thorn in the flesh, but he will give you the grace to bear it:

> 'How long, O Lord? Will you forget me for ever?
> .... Look on me and answer, O Lord my God.
> .... But I trust in your unfailing love;
> my heart rejoices in your salvation
> I will sing to the Lord for He has been good
> to me.'

There is nothing to be ashamed of in crying to the Lord, and Ian and I were to learn later on that He does answer and He does bring peace. It can take a very long time and often we are brought to the point where there is only God left, to the point when we have to submit wholly to His Will and only then can he give us the grace that we need.

Practical hints for coping with spiritual depression

1 Don't lose touch with God. Complain to Him, be honest with God, yell at Him or whatever but never lose touch.
2 Read the Bible, God does speak.
Here are some starters: Psalm 13, Isaiah 29. 22-24, Luke 11. 1-11, Psalm 113, Isaiah 43. 1-5, 1 Samuel 1 and 2. 1-11.
3 Tell some other Christian, whether it is the pastor, an elder, or a friend. Share your depression and ask them to pray for you.
4 Find someone who will pray regularly with you and who will support you until you are ready to stand alone.
5 Be positive and thank God for anything and everything until you can thank God for the fleas!

7. Debate: Discussion of some Moral Issues

Moral Dilemma

I am seeking the right answer,
searching for the truth,
looking for some guidelines
questioning it all.

Is there anyone to help me
anyone to show the way.
Can you help me be objective
and tell me what is right,
help me face the issues
from tomorrow's fiction world.
These were fantasies and stories
from an author's novel dream.

How can I know the answer
I'm involved in this plight?
How can I make decisions
On the ethics of it all?

Lord I wish you would speak
Send a telegram
or phone
Paint a message on my ceiling,
Leave a note upon my door.

Every person has a comment,
Though it differs from the last.
Every Christian has a viewpoint,
Every pastor some advice.

It's alphabetti junction,
and I am all confused,
AIH, AID, HCG and all the rest.
Pergonal and Clomid,
Leased wombs or IVF.
It's time to unravel
the treatments,
the tests.

You have the solutions
To all of my dilemmas
Help me to untangle
Your morals
From our mess.

After the second miscarriage we decided that it was time for us to seek medical aid again. We were still continuing with the screening for adoption at this time, but we felt it was right to take further positive action with the medical profession.

It was after this second miscarriage that a totally dedicated Christian consultant offered to help us. He was, in fact, a member of our extended family and had not felt able to offer his help until this moment. At a time when we were very fragile, we can only thank God for His servant. Medically and spiritually, he treated us with wonderful thoroughness and gentleness. We were barren in every way at that time, but the worst thing was the spiritual barrenness.

We went to stay with this consultant for a weekend as he lived some distance from our home. He did blood and urine tests for me, to check hormone levels and a full medical examination for Ian. It was through this that he discovered that Ian had a varicocele* and referred him to a specialist. In addition, he found that my ovulatory cycles had gone completely haywire, probably due to stress and that I was low in progesterone, the hormone that sustains pregnancy.

Later that year Ian underwent an operation for his varicocele,* (the most common cause of low fertility in men). This is a small varicose vein that can cause undue pressure and reduce the sperm count. We were told that it could take three months before the effect of the operation was apparent and the sperm count increased. It seemed a comparatively short time to wait.

I was given clomiphine during the first five days of my menstrual cycle and on the 21st day an injection of HCG (Human chorionic gondotrophin)* which was to boost my hormone levels, so that if I got pregnant I would stay pregnant!

During the time that we were undergoing further tests and before the results were known, Ian and I had to face a new dilemma. As Christians, just how far were we prepared to go in accepting 'medical interference'? At that time there was no advice available for Christians suffering from infertility. However, since then the report of a working party 'Choices of Childlessness', has been published.*

The working party was set up because of a concern about the ethical implications of AIH,* AID* and other medical procedures related to conception and child-bearing. The party was set up in 1979, but the report was only published in 1982. It has particularly tried to 'provide a context of moral and theological reflection in which particular issues can be better seen for what they are and particular judgements made with a deeper insight and understanding.'[18]

As it is such a recent publication most couples we spoke to and we ourselves, had to think through the issues with no 'official' aid. Many Christians react strongly against fertility drugs, hormone injections, AIH and AID; others accept some but not all of these possibilities. Each couple has to work through the issues for themselves, taking into account general Biblical principles, other people's views, teachings by the Church leaders and so on, until they can decide together what they feel is right.

**Two other books have also been published recently. See list of references.*

Most of us admit that we will go as far as we dare to obtain a baby of our own. Alison said to me 'I would do anything, short of adultery, in order to be pregnant and have my own child.'

In the case of fertility drugs, none of the people I spoke to were given anything stronger than clomiphine. As this merely boosts the body's natural processes, much like drugs boosting insulin production in a diabetic, there does not seem to be anything morally wrong with it. There is no risk to mother or child. In my case I would not have been happy to take Pergonal as it does carry risks for the mother and the child and I would refer you to the above-mentioned report for a detailed discussion of this.

Unless one is against medical intervention in other instances there is little to be said against the use of hormone injections. Admittedly there has been some recent controversy about the use of progesterone, but this is only relevant when artificial progesterone is used. If natural progesterone is used there are no risks.

Two couples that I talked with were offered Artificial Insemination Husband (AIH). This is the simplest form of artificial insemination and there are two main areas where it can be of value. The first is where the husband's semen, though normal, cannot gain entry to the uterus. The second is where the semen is impaired, that is, the quality rather than the quantity.

In both cases AIH can be carried out in the privacy of the home and this tends to be more successful than when it has to be done under clinical conditions. Whatever the method it can impose severe tension on the couple and so it is advisable to know your own limitations and not to continue for longer than you feel happy. As Christians there seems to be little objection to the use of this method. I talked to a pastor who had been faced with a couple who had failed to conceive. Interviewing the couple, had revealed that the problem lay with the husband who was unable to maintain an erection. They were advised by the medical profession to accept AIH, as this was the only way that the husband would be able to fertilize his wife.

The couple were worried about the moral implications and had sought the advice of their pastor. He investigated the views of other clergymen before giving them advice, and between them they agreed that there was nothing wrong with this method. In fact, it was described to me as 'creative interfering'. As the pastor said, 'This method in no way interferes with the essence of marriage. It is still the union of husband and wife, albeit mechanical, and it will still be the child of both parents.'

The question of invitro fertilization (IVF) raises similar issues. Developed in Britain by Mr Patrick Steptoe and Dr Robert Edwards it was first successful and made history in 1978 with the birth of Louise Brown. It is now an established technique, most of the babies being born in Great Britain or Australia. It is a totally mechanical and artificial method of having a baby, but it is still the child of both partners.

The original use of IVF as a treatment for infertility was limited primarily to those women with damaged or diseased Fallopian tubes, which prevent an egg passing from the ovary to the uterus. More recently, its use has been extended to those women whose husbands have a very low sperm count and to some couples with unexplained infertility. It has become a 'last hope' treatment and a costly one at that. At the moment, the success rate of IVF is conveniently clouded over because of different methods between centres. However, it is estimated at between 10-20%.

The basic principles of the techniques are simple, the actual practical application is complicated, artificial and doomed to disappointment, because of the numerous hitches that can occur in the programme resulting in failure to produce an alive and very much wanted baby.

Briefly and simply the wife enters hospital just before ovulation. One or more eggs are taken from the ovary and each is transferred to a test-tube containing the ideal chemical nutrients (hence the phrase test-tube babies, coined by the press). The husband produces a semen sample from which the sperm are extracted and incubated. To each test-tube, containing one of the wife's eggs, a sample of these sperm are introduced so that fertilization can take place. The fertilized egg is incubated to allow it to start dividing and then inserted into the mother's womb. Everybody breathlessly waits to see whether the embryo (or embryos), will implant and pregnancy occur.

This apparently simple procedure raises a whole host of social, ethical and legal questions, neglected until quite recently. In 1982 a Committee of Inquiry into Human Fertilization and Embryology was set up to examine the developments in the field of 'human assisted reproduction'. Their findings were published in the Warnock Report, in July 1984.[19]

One of the issues raised by the method is that of fertilization without normal sexual intercourse taking place. It is a totally mechanical union. In fact, it could be said to be a totally 'sterile' union!

Is it right to take a human egg and a human sperm and join them together in a test-tube, creating a new human being? Some people feel that this is so 'unnatural' that it cannot have been intended by God and is therefore wrong. Others feel that the answer is not so simple. From the physical viewpoint, the removal of an egg by general anaesthesia and laparoscopy can have risks for the mother. For the baby conceived in a test-tube, there is no evidence that being outside the natural environment, even for the space of two days has any adverse effect. For the father there is no obvious risk.

On the face of it the procedure is relatively safe and for those who accept AIH it would appear to be equally acceptable as a method of treatment for infertility resulting in the birth of a child who is the product of both husband and wife.

Sadly the issue is not so clear cut. One of the problems is that it is common practice to cause superovulation in the mother by use of drugs so that several eggs are available for collection. These eggs are all fertilized so that more than one embryo can be transferred to the mother to increase the chances of success. Some of the embryos produced will not be used—they are 'spare human beings'.

What should be done with these 'spares'? There are three options at this stage. 1. Discard the excess and allow it to die. 2. Freeze it for use at a later stage, either by its own genetical parents or by donation to another couple. 3. Allow the embryo to grow and use it for research.

If it is to be destroyed, is this the wilful destruction of life as many Catholics believe? Does anyone have the right to create new life knowing that it will probably never reach its potential?

If it is to be frozen, is this really safe and if so for how long? Who has the right to decide on the care and future use of the 'spare embryo': its genetical parents or the medical body that removed and stored it?

If it is to be subjected to medical experimentation, what 'rights' does the human embryo have? How much will we allow to be done to the embryo using the excuse that research will improve the treatment of infertility in the future? How long may an embryo be kept alive? Will we start manufacturing embryos purely for the sake of research? Possible exploitation of the embryo raises the same kinds of problem that occur in experimentation on aborted embryos. Detailed discussion of the subject goes beyond the scope of this book, but as Christians we should be involving ourselves in this subject before it becomes a fait accompli. What's more, those of us considering IVF treatment should be absolutely sure where we stand on this matter, it may be your potential offspring who is to go under the microscope next.

The Warnock report has produced firm recommendations for legislation to prevent exploitation beyond a certain level. Principally it supports IVF treatment and licensed experimentation on human embryos up to fourteen days old, with the consent of the genetic parents whenever possible.[20]

One couple who are at present seeking help through a private clinic have very kindly agreed to share their story. Meredith and Keith have been trying to have a baby for five years and have been right through the medical check-system. The hospital concentrated on Meredith who was found to have several malfunctions. These were treated by drugs and by surgery. Finally she was given a clean bill of health but still she didn't conceive. Eventually they decided to check Keith and he was found to have a very low sperm count! He has undergone surgery for a massive varicocele, which has resulted in a marked improvement. Yet still there is no baby.

Time is against them, because Meredith is 31 and has been told that her age is going to restrict their choices and chances. 'We want to have a family. In the eyes of society we are only a couple. After all, everyone talks about 'trying to have a family'. Well, we can try and try and we can wait and wait, hoping that Keith's sperm count will rise to a satisfactory level. Yet, in the end of the day, if we cannot have our own child we would like to adopt. That's where the snag lies, because once I reach 35, I cannot adopt.'

Meredith and Keith have reached a 'last chance, last fling' situation. They cannot afford the time to wait and their GP has strongly advised them to act now. They have just been accepted for IVF due to their long medical history and 'advancing' age!

'I have got to try everything,' said Meredith 'because this is my greatest desire—to have a baby. I admit that it has become an obsession with me. However, I won't go to any lengths, I will draw the line if they can't get an egg or enough live sperm. We want our baby. IVF is natural in the sense that although it uses medical methods it produces our baby. Just because our bodies don't function as they should, why should I be denied the chance to have my own child, as though it were my own fault?'

After much prayer and heart-searching Keith and Meredith are both convinced that this is right for them. Yet they have received very mixed reactions from Christian friends. Some are genuinely delighted that they have one more chance. Others are frankly critical and hurtful in their comments. 'As a Christian you shouldn't have this obsession' or 'If God wanted you to have a baby it would have happened naturally' . . Comments such as these have caused Meredith to withdraw because she doesn't want to 'feel like a freak'. She and her husband have prayed about their decision. She said, 'I have come to the point where I believe IVF is right for us, otherwise I wouldn't be doing it. We are going to go ahead and if we have mistaken God's will then it just won't work. This is my only chance, my last hope.'

The IVF programme raises expectations high, perhaps unfairly since the success rate is so low. It is long-winded and very expensive yet it has an irresistible lure because of its futuristic methods. It fascinates and draws the media and therefore the public. If the egg could be fertilized in the fallopian tube, using a laparoscopy technique, it wouldn't be a test-tube baby and there would be no glamour. Perhaps we need some of that in a last chance attempt.

In reality it is a very stressful programme, available only to a minority of rigidly screened couples. Anyone seriously contemplating it should seek medical and spiritual counselling and take time to consider its full implications. For many there will be other alternatives, which will be preferable.

The methods that raise serious moral objections are IVF with egg donation; IVF with embryo donation; AID; surrogate motherhood and womb leasing.

Egg donation is useful as a method of treatment for those women who cannot produce a viable egg. The procedure is the same as previously explained, except that instead of the wife producing her own egg, she receives a donor egg, which has been fertilized by her husband's sperm, in a test-tube.

The procedure is complex, because at the moment freezing and thawing of viable eggs is unsuccessful. Therefore, an egg must be used as soon as it is collected. This means that a donor must reach her ovulation time simultaneous to the recipient woman reaching hers. Thus, two women have to be closely monitored and this further reduces the chances of success.

Due to the difficulties of timing, it would be quite complex to have to match donor eggs, for example with respect to eye colour. The most that could be expected would be to match ethnic origin and check genetic health.

The Warnock committee accepted egg donation as a recognized treatment for infertility, although they commented on the risk taken by the donor.[21] This is a physical risk due to general anaesthesia, laparoscopy and the possibility of introduction of infection. The best method is to remove 'spare' eggs from a woman who is undergoing IVF herself and has superovulated, since this woman is already undergoing surgery.

Egg donation has one advantage over AID. In this case the husband donates the sperm and the wife incubates the resulting embryo. Thus both partners share in the production of the baby.

Embryo donation on the other hand, is where neither parent contributes genetically, both the egg and the sperm are donated. It can be used for the small minority of women who cannot produce their own eggs and whose husbands are also infertile. It is really 'pre-natal adoption', the benefit lying in the fact that once the embryo is successfully transplanted, the pregnancy is theirs. The woman can enjoy the experience of pregnancy whilst the husband observes and partakes in the joy of development like any other prospective father. He can be present at the birth like any natural father and from the moment of birth the baby is theirs with no further pressures from outside. Mechanical interference only occurs at the start of the pregnancy and they can limit who knows that the baby is not genetically theirs. In adoption any onlooker can observe the arrival of a baby or child overnight.

Embryo donation may seem ideal, especially in the present climate, where adoption of healthy white babies is so difficult. However, it is not without social, moral and legal implications, the scope of which is beyond this book. The main issues are risk to the female donor, complication of achieving a successful pregnancy without excessive medical interference and cost, the social implications of genetic record when a baby is recorded as the natural child of its adoptive parents, the legal implications should a donor wish to change his mind and so on. The Warnock committee accepted IVF and its attendant issues and therefore felt duty bound to accept egg donation and embryo donation.[22]

As a Christian it might be pertinent to question whether pre-natal adoption is really as acceptable as post-natal adoption. If as a couple you are unable to produce your own egg and your own sperm, then you cannot have your own genetic child. The arguments for experiencing pregnancy and birth, or for producing an adoptive baby when babies are so short requires minute scrutiny. Is this a justifiable use of time and money? If not, there really are hundreds of children who need a loving Mum and Dad.

The other three methods of treatment, AID, surrogate motherhood and womb leasing, involve one partner.

In the first, AID, the wife is impregnated artificially by the semen of a carefully screened, but unknown donor, usually because the husband is infertile, although it can be used to avoid hereditary disease. The donor is screened for genetic disorders and then is matched ethnically and by blood group to the woman. In some parts of the country AID is available on the National Health Service, as well as in private clinics and it is believed that many thousands of babies are born by this method every year, although valid statistics are unavailable due to the anonymity and secrecy of the procedure at present.

Before discussing the moral objections to this method, let me come back to the personal level. I have found very few Christian couples willing to admit that they have seriously considered this and to date have found no couple who have accepted it. Two women, however, did share their stories with me and they were very honest about their feelings.

Deborah learned soon after her marriage that her husband was completely sterile and that they would therefore be unable to have children of their own. Nevertheless she did not believe that they would never have a child because she had been assured that God planned a child for them. This meant one of three things; miraculous healing for her husband; AID; or adoption. The question of AID was the one that caused the problem. Deborah told me: 'My husband and I discussed it together and he was completely against it in principle. He felt that it was morally wrong for Christians and that put an end to it. You can't go ahead with something as difficult as AID unless both partners are completely happy. Maybe if I had had to make the decision myself I too would have decided that it was not right, but as it is I do feel rather differently. You see, I would like to 'grow' a baby. To me it would be like giving birth to an adoptive baby and I would have known the joy of pregnancy and motherhood. To be really honest I would do anything to have a baby, so long as it wasn't immoral.'

That was the crunch for them. Her husband believed that it was immoral and although her heart told her something different, Deborah was able to accept his view. Later we talked about surrogate motherhood and I asked Deborah how she would have felt if she had been sterile. Would she have wanted her husband to have a child by 'another woman'? 'You've really got me there. I've never thought it out but my initial reaction is that I wouldn't like it one bit!'

The second person shared with me through a letter. Miriam is in her thirties and had been married a long time before they discovered that due to childhood illness her husband would never be able to father a child. She had the same three choices as Deborah, but there the similarity ends. Miriam did not want to consider AID, her husband was all for it. He wanted her to experience the joy of pregnancy, he would prefer to adopt a baby that was his wife's although not his, rather than adopt a child that belonged to neither of them. Miriam wrote:

'I did go to an AID clinic three times, however, I wasn't very happy about it and so I stopped going. My husband was, and still is very keen and this causes some tension between us. I feel I am being mean to deny him this opportunity of having a baby in this seemingly natural way, especially when my feelings are rather confused.

I feel that if I had a baby by AID, then for the rest of my life I would be living a lie. It has to be kept a secret and I don't think I could cope with the deception. I also feel it would or could damage my relationship with God—having this secret I could never admit to. Before God it seems rather adulterous to me.

Another problem is that of Christian friends. Many of them know a bit about our problem. What if I was suddenly to become pregnant? Everyone would be giving praise and thanks to God for a miracle and it would all be a lie. The only alternative would be to tell the truth and that is impossible.

Then there is the question of the baby itself. I don't want just anybody's child. I want my husband's child because I love him. If it can't be his then I don't really want to know. Also, I would rather that both our relationships to the baby were equal, either that we are both natural parents or that neither of us are.

There is just one other point, I believe that God can change this situation.'

Miriam went on to say that when she went to the AID clinic she did not receive any kind of counselling, either medical or spiritual. It would appear to be as easy to obtain as an abortion and the amount of counselling depends upon the scruples of the individual medical practitioner.

Miriam went on to say, 'I absolutely hated the AID clinic. I don't think I have ever felt so degraded or unclean.' This is a common reaction in women and is not confined to AID clinics. Many women feel this way about the whole medical procedure and this is another reason why each couple must make their own decision about how far they personally are prepared to go, over and above the moral issues.

I have always felt that I, personally could not accept AID, because like Miriam I did not want 'another man's' child, I wanted Ian's child. I felt that the joy of pregnancy would be diminished by the knowledge that it was not my husband's baby, but that of someone unknown. Having been pregnant, I know that there is fulfilment in the purely physical changes that occur in pregnancy. As I changed in shape Ian was excited with me, he had a real pride in my bulging body, he had a possessiveness about me and the baby growing within me and I in turn was thrilled by his joy. Obviously the pleasure that we experienced through my pregnancy was just a little more acute because we had to wait so long and had begun to give up hope. Had the baby growing within me belonged to some other man, I sincerely believe that there would have been a shadow case, a third person whose presence was unwanted yet would hang around.

Ian and I discussed AID at length, before we knew the reason for our infertility and even at that time, when there was the possibility that medical investigations might show this to be the only way we could have a child of our own, I knew that it would be unacceptable. The moral issues have always daunted me.

The first and most serious objection raised, in my opinion, is the breaking of the marriage vows, which we make before God. When we marry we promise to 'love, comfort, honour and keep (each other) in sickness and in health'. Infertility can be described as 'sickness' in the same way that heart, liver, kidney, stomach malfunctions can be described as 'sickness'. Malfunction of the reproductive system is surely no different from malfunction of any other organ. This being the case Ian and I promised to love, comfort, honour and keep each other under these circumstances—and that meant accepting each other as we were. If it had turned out that Ian had been physically unable to give me a child, then surely by my marriage vows I was bound to accept him as he was and therefore accept the consequences. I could not and still cannot see that if my desire to bear a child was so great that I would be prepared to bear another man's child, that this would be honouring to Ian and it certainly would not be comforting to him.

Miriam raised the question of whether it is adulterous or not. I have asked many clergymen and Christians about this and the general feeling is that the practice is not actually adulterous, since it does not involve any form of relationship with the other man. It is purely medical treatment. However, it cannot be said to be 'hallowing of the union between man and woman', which is another of the ordinances of marriage.

Marriage was also ordained for 'the companionship, help and comfort which husband and wife ought to have of each other. It is possible that AID might threaten this. The child that is born will have an unequal relationship with its parents. With the child's mother there will be the relationship of flesh and blood, with the father it will be that of adoption. This is not to say that adopted children are not loved and cherished by their parents, but it is acknowledged that even in a re-marriage situation, the step-parent has a different relationship than the blood parent, with each child.

It has not yet been possible to investigate the long-term effects of AID, but it would seem reasonable to suppose that there will come a time in most marriages where the strain of caring for your children puts undue pressure on the individual partners. In this instance, it is quite reasonable to suppose that there might be a feeling of 'my' child and 'your' child. However temporary or fleeting the thought this will give unbearable pressure to the couple.

Infertility in itself can cause the breakdown of marriages, because of the pressure that it exerts. You have only to pick up a copy of CHILD's newsletter to read numerous heartbreaking accounts of marriage breakdowns and in some cases divorce. Christian marriages are under considerable strain today and it cannot be assumed that Christians are immune from this particular pressure. A Baptist minister's wife told me 'Infertility makes or breaks marriages,' and she was talking about Christians.

To a man, sterility is devastating. It knocks at his manhood in a way that we women find hard to comprehend. When it hits him, he is going to need all the companionship, help and comfort that his wife can give him. The stigma that he feels will stay with him for the rest of his life, even if it is subdued most of the time. Surely at times of depression this feeling will be exacerbated by the child that is his and yet not his. He will be reminded that he could not give his wife a child, that another man, an unknown man had to do it.

There comes a time for all of us when we have to accept the consequences of whom we have married. Dr James Dobson clearly holds this view, as can be seen from his books and lectures, but more particularly in his latest book '*Straight Talk To Men And Their Wives*'[23], in which he makes it plain that we choose to marry one person for life. He points out that there are some things we must learn to accept in our partners, because we can never change them, and that we must do this, not grudgingly and pointedly, but willingly and silently. If it is too difficult to accept on our own, than as Christians we can go to our Lord and seek His support and help.

This concept is true, whether we are talking about an irritating habit, an unpleasant characteristic or a physical malfunction. As Dobson points out some women have to accept that their husbands will never be able to satisfy their romantic desires and although this may seem a small point in comparison with infertility this is by no means so. A wife and mother needs to be respected and appreciated by her husband and if he cannot satisfy this longing then she lives with her unfulfilled needs every day of her life. Dobson shows that this can lead to low self-esteem, total depression and in many cases marital breakdown.

This is an example of a psychological need that some men cannot meet because of the way God made them. They are incapable of ever fulfilling their wife's desires. In the same way some men cannot meet the physical need of giving their wife a baby. She too has to live with this for the rest of her life and she too must be willing to accept the man God has given her. No-one has a perfect husband, or a perfect wife for that matter, each of us has to learn to honour the vows that we made before God, to love and to cherish until death us do part and if that means accepting a husband, or wife's sterility, then we must seek God's grace to do so.

To me these have always been the most important bars to AID, (and to egg donation) however there are others which are equally disturbing. At present there is total confidentiality with regard to donor and recipient. This means two things; the child has an unknown identity and the father has an unknown child.

Let us look first at the father. At present there are no legal restrictions on how often a donor's sperm may be used for AID, although many clinics have set individual standards. Yet it is still feasible that any one donor could be father to numerous children. A genetic history is usually kept by the individual clinics (though some clinics destroy their records once a pregnancy is achieved, in the cause of anonymity) and this, plus the restriction on how often a man may be a donor, should serve to prevent undesirable conceptions in the future. If the recommendations of the Warnock report are accepted then legislation will be brought in to ensure that inadvertent incestuous relationships do not occur.[24]

Even so each donor may have several unknown children. As Christians we believe that marriage was ordained for 'the welfare of human society' God ordained that a man and a woman should be bound irrevocably together, in love and respect for one another. From their love children should be conceived and within the marriage unit a family be formed. Mother and father should have the unique responsibility for the upbringing of their offspring, physically, emotionally and spiritually.

AID disrupts this God-given plan, for the biological father cannot also be the social father. Once the donor has played his part, he has no further knowledge of or interest in his offspring. He cannot take any responsibility for the child's life, he is merely a tool in its creation.

For the Christian man donorship is surely an impossibility. He is denied his God-given responsibility for his child. He can never insist that the child is given spiritual training, he will never know if his child is physically or emotionally maltreated. The Christian donor cannot insist that the recipients are Christians and he cannot be sure that the home will be one that he would want his child brought up in.

At present the recommendations of the Warnock report are that at eighteen a child should legally have access to information about his genetic father; ethnic origin and genetic health only, so that anonymity is preserved.[25] It is, however, just conceivable that in the future, as with adoption, the child will be permitted access to his files in order to establish his ancestry. Can you even begin to imagine the situation where a donor is suddenly confronted with one, two, three or possibly many more adolescents or young adults whom he has fathered? What responsibility emotional, spiritual or physical can this father now take for his children, all of whom have different mothers? What will be the feelings of the children all confronted with an assortment of step-brothers or sisters? The situation is farcical and would be uproarously funny on stage, but what of real life?

So we return to the biological mother, the social father and his child. If the true facts are never disclosed it can be argued that the child will not suffer. Yet do we not accept that genetic ancestry plays an important part in the characteristics of an individual? And what of the parents who have to hold this secret for life?

Jesus said: '. . . I am the Truth . . .' (John 14. 6) and as Christians we seek to be like Jesus. The psalmist says, 'Surely you (God) desire truth in the inner parts;' (Psalm 51. 6 NIV). We are commanded to be truthful; 'These are the things you shall do: Speak the truth to one another, render in your gates judgements that are true and make for peace.' (Zechariah 8. 16 RSV)

How can we, who are called to truthfulness, live a lie for the rest of our lives? As with all lies, this one has several facets. First there is the lie to the child, he is not in truth his 'father's' child. Second there is the lie to our family and friends, people who trust us, and this attacks the value of these relationships. Thirdly, for those who have Christians praying for their infertility, it requires a more serious deceit, that of allowing those Christians to believe that God has healed and has given a 'miracle' child. How will the couple, and more particularly the father, cope when they hear thanks and praise being given to God for a child who is in fact only half theirs?

Lastly, it requires lying to the state, which by its very nature is illegal. By law it is required that both the father and mother's names are entered on the birth certificate of a child. In this case the biological father's name is unknown. If the space is left blank, firstly, by law, this will make the child illegitimate and secondly when the child is older and given his birth certificate the truth will have to be told. This revelation brings with it all the psychological problems that adoptive children once faced. To guard against this and also because at present AID is a questionable practice most people enter the social father's name. This not only messes up genetic records but is illegal.

If you decide that you will be truthful about the father's name and allow your child to be illegitimate, you will have to decide that from the moment of birth this is an open secret. Relatives and close friends will know the truth and so the child will have to be told fairly early on, as with an adoptive child. But the information you have to give him will be limited and how will he react? How will the father's parents feel about their 'grandchild'? How will the maternal grandparents react? What possible problems might the child face at school? These and endless other questions face those who decide to be open and honest about the child's conception.

It is interesting that in 1948 the Archbishop of Canterbury recommended that AID should be a criminal offence. Yet it was not until 1960 that the Feversham Committee was set up by the government to consider AID. The conclusion was that 'the majority within both society and the medical profession was opposed to the practice of AID'[26] and that it should be 'strongly discouraged'. The practice, however, continued to grow. Finally in 1971 the British Medical Association asked Sir John Peel to look into the medical aspects of AI. He recommended that AID should be available on the NHS at accredited centres. To date no system of accreditation has been established.

Today hundreds of live births take place as a result of AID and yet it is only now that the legal aspects are being seriously considered. The Warnock committee, recognizing many of the difficulties still pertinent to AID, have recommended that the child should in law be treated as the legitimate child of its mother and her husband, so that the father is registered as the father and that the biological father should have no parental rights or duties in relation to the child.[25]

As a theological or moral discussion the odds would appear to be heavily loaded against Christians conceiving by AID, but it is a purely theoretical discussion and leaves out the human element. As with divorce, about which Jesus left specific instructions, abortion, infanticide and euthanasia about which He did not specifically comment because they were not in question at the time, there is no single and simple answer which governs all cases. Each of us must face the Lord and seek his will for us as individuals. We must apply basic biblical principles, we must seek guidance and spiritual counselling, we must test and try the answers we are given and in the final analysis, each couple and each individual within the couple must make their own decision.

Surrogate motherhood and womb leasing raise even greater moral objections than AID. The arguments against AID, hold true for both these situations, but there are other issues involved as well.

Surrogacy can be used in several different ways. In its simplest form it is used for a couple where the wife is totally infertile. The husband provides the sperm, through AID and the surrogate mother provides the egg and bears the child, with the aim that at birth the child should be handed over to its adoptive mother and genetic father. A sort of pre-arranged adoption.

Alternatively, the wife may be able to produce eggs but be unable to carry a pregnancy to term, either through risk to herself or the baby. In this case she provides the egg. The sperm may be that of her husband or a donor, who is sometimes the surrogate mother's husband. The technique of IVF is used to establish the pregnancy in the surrogate mother who acts as a human incubator. This is commonly called 'womb-leasing'.

Although it is theoretically possible to have any combination of persons involved to produce a medley of genetic mother, commissioning mother, surrogate mother, genetic father, social father, commissioning husband, surrogate husband and so on, in fact, the most common is that of the surrogate mother donating the egg and carrying the baby to term and the commissioning husband donating the sperm, thus also being the genetic father. In many cases the surrogate mother is known to the commissioning couple, so there is not the same secrecy.

We read in Genesis of a threesome who tried to have a family and it didn't work out too happily.

> 'Now Sarai, Abram's wife had borne him no children. But she had an Egyptian maidservant named Hagar; so she said to Abram, 'The Lord has kept me from having children. 'Go, sleep with my maidservant; perhaps I can build a family through

her.' Abram agreed to what Sarai said . . . . He slept with Hagar and she conceived. When she knew she was pregnant, she began to despise her mistress.' Genesis 16. 1, 2, 4 (NIV)

Sarah went on to blame Abram and eventually after her own son Isaac was born she sent Hagar and Ishmael away. It is easy to imagine the kind of tensions that can build up between the partners if they are known to each other, despite the fact that today it is so clinical.

In the case of sisters, how will the infertile sister feel when she sees the child that is half her husband and half her fertile sister? Will she always feel that decisions about the child's upbringing must be made to fit in with the genetic mother's views? How will the genetic mother feel when her child is criticized by its adoptive mother? What if the adoptive mother were to die? Who would have the greater claim, the genetic father or the genetic mother? How will the child feel when it discovers that 'Auntie' is actually 'Mummy'? Surrogate motherhood between friends or relatives could ruin relationships and create a bizarre hereditary maze.

The difficulty with surrogacy is that the donor's part lasts for forty weeks. During these weeks the future 'parents' have little involvement; the husband gives his sperm for the insemination, they wait anxiously for the outcome, a pregnancy is achieved, they wait again, this time until the baby is due. It is only at this point when the baby is born that they both become actively involved, when, in fact they take 'their' baby.

The donor woman carries the baby for nine months and her involvement with the foetus will vary with the individual. Some women have a pride in what they are doing, they enjoy pregnancy (a mother once told me that the only time she felt completely healthy and vital was when she was pregnant, but that she could not afford to keep having babies. This method of motherhood would be ideal!) According to a television programme some women have a real joy in knowing that they can give an infertile couple a child that is half theirs and because of this they have the same excitement and anticipation that they would have with their own child. The husbands of the donors also become involved in this feeling, which makes up for some of the inconvenience of having a pregnant wife!

Unfortunately there are others who do it for the money, and the fee is good. (Although one woman said that when you divide the fee by 40 weeks it works out at a very low income for the amount of involvement.) Some husbands are cautious of their wives 'selling' their bodies this way, feeling it to be degrading.

Motherhood in this sense is very questionable. Some would call it mercenary. It can be very clinical. And what of the child? Could it be humiliating to the child to know it has been 'bought'? What of the relationship between surrogate mother and child? Nowadays much stress is laid on the relationship built between the mother and the foetus from the early days. In most cases the mother goes on to look after that same baby. Do we know how it affects the baby to be removed from the woman that has nurtured it and given to another woman? Is it right to voluntarily do this to a newborn infant? What of the pregnancy itself?

The social mother has no influence over the behaviour of the biological mother. She cannot dictate how much alcohol, coffee, drugs are taken. Whose responsibility is it if a child is affected from some drug inadvertently taken? Whose responsibility is it if the child is born handicapped—will the social mother be able to accept the child? Who takes the decision if antenatal tests show that the foetus has spina bifida? Whose responsibility is it if there is a miscarriage?

What of the risks attached to pregnancy? Supposing the surrogate mother changes her mind and decides to keep the baby? If the surrogate mother kept the baby, could she later claim an affiliation order on the genetic father?

Even though it might be an act of generosity on the part of the donor and a last chance for the couple, there are even more unanswered questions in this method than in AID. It has been said that 'Surrogate motherhood is hardly motherhood at all.'[3]

With respect to womb-leasing it could be argued that this method is preferable to surrogate motherhood because the involvement of the 'donor' is purely physical since it is not her child and that it does not break the vows of marriage because the resultant child will belong to both parents. However many of the questions raised above still apply, such as regulating the pregnancy. In addition there is bound to be an anxiety factor for the biological parents who have given their joint child to a 'foster' mother and they cannot be involved for nine months. What will be the maternal feelings of the biological mother?

It is also a very complex method if two women both have to be brought to the correct phases of their menstrual cycle at the same time.

One other factor that is sometimes raised relates also to AID. In the latter case it is possible for a single woman to have a child by artificial insemination. This does not involve the sex act, but does give her the chance of a pregnancy and motherhood. A recent TV report called 'The American Documentary' showed that at least in America some women are seeking this alternative. One woman said that as so many marriages break up and the child is left without a father anyway, it would be better for the child to start off with only a mother!

In womb-leasing it is feasible that a couple could have a child, without the mother having the 'bother' of a nine-month pregnancy. For a career woman this would give her another nine months freedom, another nine months income before the burden of the child. Is it possible that such an horrific thing could ever happen? People didn't believe in test-tube babies, either. In fact, the Warnock Committee have recommended that all forms of surrogacy should be made illegal.[27]

As trends in society mean that infertility is on the increase it is logical that more research will be done into the treatment of infertility. The increasing awareness of the plight of infertile couples, brought about largely by the self-help groups, means that more money is becoming available and more researchers and doctors are becoming interested in this subject.

Already our country and more especially Christians are

facing legal and moral questions that our grandparents didn't even have nightmares about. It is time that we made our decisions on the present issues and that we prepare ourselves to face the future.

As Christians we do not have only ourselves to consider. There comes a time when we not only accept the consequences of our choice of marriage partner, but we must also face our commitment to God. It may be that however much we want a child, there are some practices which are not and in the future will not be permissible to us. It may be that we will have to accept the undeniably hard facts and stand out against some of the present and future practices.

It is no easy task but we have a power beyond ourselves which enables us to accept the unacceptable.

Practical hints on dealing with moral issues

1. Make your decisions while you can still be objective, that is before you are in the swing of medical tests.
2. Talk to other Christians, whether or not they have similar problems. Badger your pastor, elders, and other spiritual leaders. Weigh up their replies against the principles of scripture.
3. When it comes to the major issues remember that both of you must be 100% happy about the decision. You cannot even contemplate AID, for example, if one partner has misgivings.
4. Read 'Why US?' by Dr Stanway. A secular book but it deals in detail with many of the moral issues.
5. When you have done your research, go away for a long weekend. Talk together. Pray together. Seek the Lord. Then make your decision and stand by it.

8. Contentment: Our Total Submission

Total Surrender

Like Houdini I've been chained
By my will
By my choice
Locked in a death trap
Held in an unyielding vice.

But you in your loveliness
You in your grace
Gave me the chance to rise and escape
I had forgotten the combination
I was dying by myself
But you in your mercy let me fly free.

You are my sovereign
You are my king
You have the right
To everything
I am learning to yield
To submit my will
To bend the knee
Prayerfully.

Total submission
Total surrender
Total relief
Total peace

Teach me your ways, Lord
I'd know your mind
Daily come closer.

Released from my bondage
Your glory
I see
I can rejoice
Give praise
Give thanks

Your will, not mine
I now have the key.

We came home to await the results of the latest series of tests carried out and while we waited we took some sound advice. It is a well-known fact that many couples conceive whilst on a really relaxing holiday. What a wonderful excuse to go abroad and live it up and that is exactly what we did! In June we spent two idyllic weeks in Italy, perspiring in the hot sunshine, soaking up culture until we were saturated with Michelangelo, stuffing pastas and ice-cream like only Mama used to make.

We 'did' Rome and Pompeii and then sank exhausted into deckchairs under a sunshade protecting our lily white English bodies from the cruel midday sun and enviously watching the brown-skinned Italians at play. We swam, hiked, shopped and totally immersed ourselves in another world for fourteen glorious days. But we didn't get pregnant.

When we arrived home there was a letter waiting for Ian, inviting him for a job interview in two days time. Refreshed and relaxed, he went along and to our astonishment got it. We were thrilled.

I gave up my job and decided to try a spell as a housewife, since many doctors believe that this can be a psychological trigger and it was one of the methods we had not yet tried. New horizons opened up for us; a new job, a new town, a new church. As we prepared for all these changes, God was thawing our hearts. How patient He is.

In our new locality we became aware of how richly and unexpectedly God blesses. We found a lovely fellowship and a Christian group practice with a wonderful GP, who has since become a very dear friend. Ian's new job was a great thrill to him, to such an extent that he bemoaned the weekends as an interruption to his exciting weeks! I, in turn, settled happily into the role of being a housewife and enjoyed a new creativity, experimenting with knitting, embroidery and sewing (none of which I have mastered, but it was fun trying!) I began to learn the fast-fading art of homemaking.

Whilst all these things were going on, our application for fostering had been grinding its way around the system. We were so busy with the move that we had almost forgotten about it until one day, a month after we moved we had a phone call to say that we had been accepted as long-term foster parents. Then a few days later came the bomb-shell, they had a baby for us. We were offered a four-month-old baby boy with galactosaemia*. I was in the middle of taking the vacuum cleaner apart to mend it (new horizons!) when the call came and afterwards I was shaking so much that I couldn't get the screws back in the correct holes.

As it happened we had known about Benjamin from his birth. During one of our questioning sessions the social worker had mentioned this new baby that had come on their books, because his illness was of interest to me. We had thought no more about it, but it seemed that the mother had dallied about whether to put him up for adoption. At last she had made the decision and we had simultaneously been accepted for fostering.

The timing was perfect, or so it seemed to us. To the social services, we were the right couple because I was a dietician and had been working in a childrens' hospital and in addition, the mother had specifically asked that the child should be taken by Christian parents. So the thing that had held up our acceptance by the social services was now the very thing that had got us a baby so quickly. It truly seemed like the Lord at work!

It was love at first sight when we saw Ben. His smile was totally captivating and he was so cuddly. We held him, fed him, played with him for a whole afternoon and the social worker and temporary foster mother both remarked that we fitted like two pieces of jigsaw. We were captivated and yet wary. We wanted Ben, yet we shied away from the enormity of it all. This was no light-hearted venture, Ben was up for adoption. This was for life. It held all the awe of marriage, an unbreakable covenant.

We prayed earnestly and at the back of our minds was the fact that if this went ahead then it might be God's way of telling us that we would never conceive. We were torn by our emotions. In truth a part of us was not quite ready for this step. Being at home I was able to spend time seeking the Lord. When we were engaged to be married, I had agonized before the Lord for fear of making the wrong decision and I did so again now. I earnestly wanted to do His will. I had learned that to step out of His way was to court disaster and real unhappiness, and conversely to walk with God was to be at peace.

Preparations for taking Ben home proceeded swiftly. I wanted Ben more and more and in seeking the Lord I unconsciously looked for confirmation. One morning I turned on the radio and heard the story of Isaac and Ishmael. It seemed that God was telling me that first we would have another woman's child and then our own. It was the same story that had spoken to me earlier in the year, in which I had received the promise that I would bear a child. Now it seemed logical and right that we should adopt first.

Everything seemed so right except for one small point. Ben was rather slow in his physical responses. We knew that galactosaemia could affect the mental ability of a child, but this physical aspect was rather surprising. We went to see his paediatrician, who was very encouraging, although he didn't have Ben's notes with him. He remembered the baby and could see little to worry about, howeve he did agree to do a full routine check-up before we took Ben home.

I went with the foster mother to the hospital and was present while the paediatrician carried out a thorough examination. Afterwards we went into his office and this time he had the medical notes as well. He was gravely disturbed by Ben's lack of responses. The notes revealed that Ben had been a forceps delivery and that he had taken fifteen minutes to breathe. All these factors set alarm bells ringing in my head and I wished fervently that Ian could have been with me.

He wasn't, so I began to question the doctor about the prognosis. He was reticent. He would not give an opinion, but slowly it became apparent that he thought Ben was both physically and mentally handicapped. I requested a second opinion and asked that he be referred to Great Ormond Street.

By the time I got home, I was really confused. The foster mother and social worker did not believe the doctor, but I was beginning to open my eyes. The medical information was enough to tell me that something was seriously wrong. That evening I phoned my parents, they advised extreme caution and admitted to having had some grave doubts (my mother had come with me on one of my visits to Ben and it was she who had remarked on his lack of response). I phoned the chief dietitian at Great Ormond Street, who was both a friend and a dedicated Christian. She gave me the statistics regarding galactosaemia and mental retardation illustrating that the picture was much blacker than I had first realized.

Everything had been going so smoothly that I couldn't believe it was going wrong now. I had grown accustomed to the thought that we were to have Ben. He was due home in ten days and I had finally gone out and bought a whole lot of baby equipment. So what was happening? In effect I asked, what was God playing at? Why had he brought us this far? I turned to the Bible and read from Romans 14, seeking reassurance:

> 'Accept him who is weak . . . without passing judgement on disputable matters . . . he will stand for the Lord.' I drew encouragement from these words even though they were taken out of context.

How desperately I wanted this baby, my Ishmael. At first we had told no-one about Ben, but with only ten days to go, we had rung close friends and family. Already we had received one or two cards and parcels. Our joy was their joy and it was as exciting as a pregnancy. What if it all went wrong now? I was frozen with fear, yet I had learnt enough to know that I must find out God's will.

Ian and I talked and prayed. Alone I beseeched the Lord to be clear. But it was not clear. As doubts rose within me, so did the panic. This was commitment for life. Three of us would be closely involved and many others would be affected. How would Ian's mother feel when we told her that we were adopting a child who would certainly be mentally retarded and maybe even physically handicapped? She was completely against what we were doing anyway. My parents were seriously worried. Close friends were cautious and divided in their opinion.

I came back before the Lord, willing to admit my helplessness; to admit that I had been making scripture say what I wanted it to and to ask His help. I prayed that if we were wrong, that God would slam the door in our faces, even if He caught our fingers and it hurt.

Next day I went to Great Ormond Street. Ian could not get time off work, so my father came with me. The foster mother came with Ben. We had to be there by nine o'clock, because the consultant was leaving for the airport at ten, he wouldn't be back in England for two weeks and by then it would be too late, we would have had Ben. He had kindly squeezed us in before he left.

The examination was thorough. He was a very experienced and competent specialist. As he carried out the tests, I willed Ben to respond, but even to my inexperienced eyes I could see that he was slow. Despite his tight schedule the specialist did not hurry. He really seemed to care. At last he sat down and faced me. He did not beat about the bush. From the test he had done and the medical history it was highly probable that Ben would be both severely physically and mentally handicapped.

'I could be wrong. I hope so, but in all fairness I don't think so. The chances that he will escape or have a mild handicap are minimal. At this stage the odds are already loaded against him. Now, of course miracles do happen. With time, patience and luck you might be able to improve on the handicap, but it is going to require total undivided care and attention for the rest of this child's life. I don't know anything about you and your husband, maybe this is for you, a child that you can dedicate your lives to. Heaven alone knows he needs someone who will love him and care for him—exclusively.'

He paused before continuing, 'I do not wish to dissuade or persuade you. It is not my job to counsel you, only to give you the medical facts, which I have done. However, I will say this. Ben needs utter commitment. You would not have time for another child. If you knew that you and your husband could never bear a child, then maybe you could choose to take Ben. However, if there is any chance that you might get pregnant, then I would urge you to think very very carefully about this. That is all the advice I can give you.'

Dad and I talked all the way home. I was reminded that we had agreed to take any child under five, of any race and with almost any problem, except severe mental and physical handicap. Dad was marvellous. He was obviously disturbed, but he assured me that the decision belonged with Ian and me. Whatever we decided, he and Mum would back us. If we turned Ben down, they would, frankly, be relieved, but they knew how disappointed we would be. If we went ahead, then they would accept Ben as their grandson and would support us in every possible way. He helped me see every angle, but he did not try to force his view onto me.

When Ian got home, I cried silently because I knew God had slammed the door and I was hurt. When my Mum 'phoned the floodgates opened and we really wept together. She was so distressed that God had let us get so close and then taken away the baby. And I, amidst my self-pity, cried for the baby who had no chance of a normal life. I felt guilty that we could not offer him the love and care that he needed, I felt that somehow I had failed and that increased my hurt. The social services told us that it might be two years before we were offered another child and we felt that this was emotional blackmail.

One week later and Ben would have been ours. We grieved bitterly that this baby, the third, had been taken away from us, but our strengthened faith stood firm in the face of this new disappointment. This time we didn't revel in our self-pity, we had asked God to clearly guide and he had. It might hurt, but it was right.

What followed was truly the refiner's fire. We now faced the question not only of no child of our own, but of no child at all. Were we willing? During the last two years we had been prepared to sacrifice our faith in God, in our desire to have children. Were we willing, in turn, to sacrifice our desires to have children, for our faith in God? If He said 'Childless', would we accept?

We had been living on a seesaw. In times of hope our faith would be strong and we would see God's hand at work but as soon as problems arose or things did not go as we had expected doubts would crowd our minds and we would be tossed about as though we had no anchor.

Now, in December 1980, we were down low. In January of the same year I had received a word that seemed to come directly from the Lord. My father had been reading from Genesis 18 during family prayers and he read these words:

> 'Then the Lord said, "I shall surely return to you about this time next year and . . . your wife will have a son".

Afterwards three members of the family spoke to me on separate occasions saying that as these words were read, they had felt the Lord speaking about me. As I had listened that morning I had also responded in this way. Throughout 1980 I had hugged this promise to me. With each fresh disappointment, with each passing month I reminded God of His words. If anything had kept me going it had been this verse and as the months passed I kept thinking that although they brought disappointment they were also bringing me closer to the promise and its fulfilment.

In November with the offer of Ben for adoption I had again heard from the story of Sarah and Abraham, in the radio service. I had been only half listening but suddenly I was fully alert and taking in every word that I heard. In my human mind I was surprised that God was giving us an adopted child in November, because that only gave Him December to fulfil His promise within me. Now in December it was too late and I was holding God to ransom. We didn't have Ishmael, God had taken him away, so what of Isaac?

I spent a long time in prayer before the Lord. By now I knew that he was in control and I knew that He had something to teach us, but what? As with the adoption of Ben I truly wanted to do His will, yet I was afraid of what God might be asking. I read again the story of Sarah and Abraham, seeing that I had misinterpreted yet looking again for a special word. As I read chapters 21 and 22 of Genesis I began to panic. First God took Ishmael from Abraham and then He asked for Isaac:

> 'Then God said (to Abraham), "Take your son, your only son Isaac, whom you love, and go to the region of Moriah. Sacrifice him there as a burnt offering on one of the mountains I will tell you about." '
>
> (Genesis 22. 2 NIV)

God asked Abraham to show his love by sacrificing his only son. Was I willing to sacrifice my promise, the promise of a child, even before his birth? Was I really willing to say 'Lord, I love you and fear you and you are more important to me than anything, even having a baby'? Was I willing to say with Jesus[25] 'Not my will but yours' however hard that is? Not for a long time.

The Lord deals patiently with His children. He does not spare those whom He loves, but rather He tries, tests, disciplines, refines them. We had had several difficulties over the past two years and the two hardest to bear were a split in our previous church for which we had unwittingly becomes the scapegoats, and our childlessness. For two years God had been testing us, trying our faith. Now I remembered that 'anyone who loves mother or father (or child) more than God is not worthy of Him' (Matthew 10. 37) I could not bargain with God, nor hold Him to ransom. So, I surrendered.

Unknown to me Ian was simultaneously facing the

same challenge. He too surrendered. Individually we had both realized that God had the right to ask anything of us. If our faith meant anything then we must be willing to be wholehearted—no exclusion clauses. For the first time, individually and together as a couple, we placed everything unreservedly, unconditionally in His hands and faced the challenge of living without children.

This was the most important turning point—our total surrender to God. Ian and I truly believe that God had brought us to this point, that this was one of His purposes during the previous two years. God has done this throughout the ages; He did it with Job, He did it with Jonah, He did it with Joni Eareckson, He did it with us and He will go on doing it. God will bring His children to the point of unconditional surrender, the process will hurt and will be different for each one but it will be for His glory.

It was just a few days after this that my first niece was born, to my sister Diane, a beautiful gift from God. Now we could rejoice wholeheartedly with the proud parents. We had peace in God.

The New Year came and went. Six weeks later I was pregnant and we knew how gracious God is. As Joni Eareckson had surrendered her 'right' to a husband, we had surrendered our 'right' to children. Now God in his generous love had given us the gift of a pregnancy. In fact, He had done it within the year from my promise.

We rejoiced with our families but otherwise we kept this precious secret to ourselves. It was too special, too miraculous, too private to share at this stage. Due to our medical history I was advised to take things very easy and so I suddenly found myself a lady of unaccustomed leisure. Nothing to do except be a human incubator,giving everything to the new life growing within me. Each new day we woke with a song in our hearts and on our lips. Halcyon days.

By ten weeks we were ready to tell the world the glad tidings. A host of angels couldn't have sung more loudly. One afternoon I sat down with my feet up and wrote joyful letters to all our friends, words tumbling gleefully onto the pages, arriving in whatever order, sentences largely incoherent and illegible as I prepared each missive. At last the letters sat in a huge tottering pile, signed, sealed and stamped—a veritable fortune ready for posting—that night I started to miscarry.

It was 5 p.m. when I realized what was happening and I sat for a while in shocked disbelief. Then my world crumbled and I was filled with unaccountable hysteria. I didn't feel angry. I knew that God has the right to give and to take away. But I was filled with intense panic. I wasn't sure that I could take this blow, I wasn't confident that I could stand the test and I wasn't sure how Ian would react. I paced the house, wandering from room to room, tears pouring unchecked down my cheeks, praying for the strength to handle this situation. In every room I looked at the clock longing for Ian to be home, hating the isolation. I wanted to lie down yet I could not stay still.

Like a child I brushed the tears away with the back of my hand. I spoke out loud and told the Lord that I would accept this also, that I knew He was sovereign, but that He would have to bear with me until I could get control of my emotions and regain my composure. I was ashamed that I couldn't stop crying and that Ian returned from work at last, to find a lump of jelly, where he should have found a peace-filled wife.

Ian was marvellous. Despite the fact he was as shaken and disappointed as I was he remained strong. He held me tight until at last the tears stopped and never once did he tell me to be more trusting. The only thing he did say was that if I didn't calm down I would lose the baby from pure hysteria! He got me into bed and when I was quiet and happy to be left he rang our GP, who accelerated into medical and spiritual action. As soon as he finished speaking to Ian he rang his wife and asked her to start praying. In turn Ian rang round our closest family, who in turn contacted their prayer partners and so a circle of prayer went into action.

Then Ian sought the Lord, opening his Bible to find a word of comfort for us. He turned to the Psalms and there he read Psalm 113. With a heavy heart he began to read and found that this is a Psalm of praise. He didn't feel all that enamoured with the idea of praising God for this situation, but he read on and when he reached verse 9 he knew the Lord had spoken.

> 'He honours the childless wife in her home; he makes her happy by giving her chldren . . . Praise the Lord.'

Ian crept into our room and found that the Lord had regained control of my emotions. As we held hands I knew the peace that passes understanding, even before Ian shared the Psalm with me. By the time our GP came order had been restored.

The doctor injected me with hormones and a heavy dose of God's love. For a week I lay flat on my back, awaiting the outcome, but it was a wonderful week. So many of our Christian friends called, loving us and supporting us by word and deed.

This was so different from the two previous occasions. This time we had totally surrendered to God and we were willing to accept his outcome. Consequently, we were able to accept the loving care offered to us. The presence of God surrounded and protected us. On the Sunday of that week the pastor preached on Psalm 113! Peace filled our hearts as we waited, it was a time of victory and we began to learn to praise the Lord.

One thing clouded those days—the tottering pile of letters still waiting to be posted. One night Ian came to me and said that he believed God wanted us to post them. I nodded, knowing that it was a confirmation of my own feelings, and watched his slow smile. It was another moment of testing, but we both knew that it was the right thing to do: to post those letters in faith.

The next night the doorbell rang. It was our pastor, who perched himself casually on the end of our bed, bringing his own special brand of encouragement. As we were chatting the doorbell rang again and minutes later the gentle smiling face of our GP appeared around the door, behind him I could see Ian's radiant one. It was good news. I was still pregnant. Together the four of us prayed, rejoicing in the Lord. What a precious moment.

Over the next few months I still had to take it easy and

I was injected weekly with Primolut*, until my twentieth week. I savoured the days of summer, having a heightened perception of life. It did me good to stop and ruminate, life had been too pressurized. Now I was filled with contentment and was happy to learn about relaxation. Ian would come home to find me lying on a sunbed, peacefully gazing at the garden, watching butterflies, listening to the sounds of life. They were some of the happiest days.

So the time passed until two weeks before the expected date of delivery. Then, because of toxaemia I had elective surgery. I was fortunate to be offered epidural anaesthesia and so I was able to be conscious throughout the caesarian. The entire team were Christians so we started with prayer and rejoiced together when our baby daughter was born. She came out assuring me that this was reality, she had finally arrived. A five pound fifteen ounce scrap of humanity, liberally covered with a coating of double cream, shouting to let all the world know that she had made it. God had given us our 'Isaac'!

[illegible] and might [illegible]
[illegible] contro[illegible]
[illegible]
[illegible] and [illegible]
[illegible]
[illegible] come [illegible] had [illegible]
[illegible]
[illegible] They were [illegible]
[illegible]
[illegible] fell in the [illegible]
[illegible]
[illegible]
[illegible]
[illegible] were [illegible]
[illegible] together [illegible]
[illegible]
[illegible] and [illegible]
[illegible] covered with [illegible]
[illegible] the [illegible]
[illegible] had made [illegible] had given [illegible]

9. Fulfilment: Accepting Childlessness

Fulfilment

Thank you
Those two simple words
Can never express
all that I want to say.
Even if I repeat them
all day
every day
for the rest of my life
they are still inadequate.

You have given me so much
my daughter
my son
Thank You
Thank You

Yet,
I am almost ashamed
I am a 'have'
no longer
a 'have-not'

This girl weeps
her husband is sterile,
What can I say?

I weep
silently
choked
heavy heart
knotted stomach.

I cannot say
'I've been there'
I haven't
But I can say
'I know'
because I have felt
the pain,
the failure,
the humiliation,
the emptiness,
the pointlessness,
the fear
the disillusionment
the despair.

Through the waiting
the 'what if . . '
I can understand
I can be there
in her experience

Yet she cannot see that
She sees only my children

I know
I feel her anger
her rebellion
I want to cry 'Why, Lord?'
but I know
there is a reason
your good reason, Lord.

I cannot help her
know you
know herself

she, alone
must accept
that you know best.

So I pray
don't push her too hard
Be quick
to comfort
Keep your promise
Fill her
Fulfil her
Soon.

Ours is a real success story. Doubly so, because since starting to write this book I have had another child—a son. God has answered our prayers beyond our expectations in that I had got to the stage of saying 'Just one, Lord, if you would only give us one child . . .'

At last we have our heart's desires, the blessings, the privileges and the problems of parenthood! We can wholeheartedly rejoice and we do daily thank God for answering our cry. In our rejoicing, in the fulfilling of our yearning we are able to look back over the struggle and to see God's hand at work. We have learnt so much through our waiting, that now we can be positive and even thank God for those years.

For some of the couples who shared their stories for this book the story is the same. If we still named our children with names that had significant meanings there would have been a sudden upsurge of Samuels[30] in the last two years! Individually and collectively we can give the praise and glory to the Lord.

But what about those couples who are still waiting—and there are many. Some of these already know that humanly speaking there is no hope, because of their medical histories, others suspect that this will be the outcome, and yet others just starting on the road dread the possibility of sterility.

Why do some couples never receive this precious, yet natural and common, gift of a child? Can Christians ever come to terms with childlessness, or infertility? Is there still a light at the end of the tunnel?

As I have talked to couples who have never and will never have a child of their own, I have come to the conclusion that there is hope. There is healing, both mental and spiritual even if God never grants physical healing. There can be peace, God can give the grace of acceptance of His will.

We all know that time dulls pain. Those who have lost loved ones know that at first the grief they experience is acute in the extreme, some people feel they cannot go on living without the partner, parent or child that they have lost. But as the days go by, the grief dulls to a constant ache which is only intensified by some incident, such as a birthday or a letter of belated sympathy which temporarily re-opens the wound. In time, the loved one, although remembered, is no longer grieved for. People do go on living, they do re-marry, they do have happy lives.

So it is with complete infertility. Most couples said that at first they had felt 'totally devastated', many had experienced a sense of disbelief, of horror at the cold finality of it all. Yet they all agreed that acceptance could and did come and that apart from the odd occasion, the agonizing at an acute level was over. Many people suffer permanent physical pain and they learn to live with it. So it is with bereavement and childlessness.

However, there is a difference between the two griefs. To quote Katherine Hall,

> 'while bereavement can be eased by the funeral rite which offers a way of taking leave of the loved one, there is no such helpful means for 'dealing with' childlessness. Even when the woman reaches the end of her child-bearing years there is no programme, no formal method of helping the couple through this very final anguish. And when death finally claims one partner, the other, with no supportive family to lean on, is alone indeed.'[28]

For the single woman the pain of childlessness becomes acute once more at the time of menopause, when she knows that even though she still has the chance to marry and spend the rest of her life with a companion, she will never be able to bear her own child. Unlike the married woman she faces this alone, unless there are those who can interpret her needs and meet them, carrying her through until acceptance has come again.

It seems to me as an onlooker, listening to others telling their stories that it was easier for those who had a suspicion of the final outcome right from the beginning.

Equally those who had adequate counselling and support from other Christians all the way along, fared much better. One lady I talked with told me: 'I was so lucky that my pastor and his wife had had a similar problem. Right from the start they supported us and right from the beginning, although they gave us sympathy they drilled it into us that God has the supreme right to do as He wills. They tutored us so that we would be ready to do whatever he wanted and they made us look positively towards the future and finding other ways to fulfil our desires for a family.'

To this day neither she nor her husband knows why they could not have children. There was no apparent medical reason. When it became obvious that they had reached the end of the road, they recognized it.

This seems to be an important factor. To be able to recognize when you can go no further, whether it is because the doctor tells you so or whether it is because you and your spouse feel that you cannot take any more of the stress and strain involved.

There comes a time when it is necessary to call a halt. Do so. Shut the door, lock it and throw away the key, because if you leave it ajar, you will be forever going back to try and prise it open again. Just one more time, just one more test, more raised hopes which will probably be dashed and the pain will be worse.

One person I spoke to said, 'I know that physically it is impossible for my husband and I to have a baby, yet I haven't really given up. I still hope that God will create a miracle and that one day I will have my own baby. Most of the time I am perfectly happy and accept my present life-style, but then something re-awakens the issue and the turmoil starts all over again. I can have really black days.'

Can it ever really be forgotten, totally and unconditionally accepted, never to ache again? I doubt it. Only one person said she had no regrets, that she was perfectly happy that she had never conceived. All the other women admitted to bad moments (husbands less so), but they all seemed to feel that it was better not to go on hoping.

It is a hard fact that God does not always answer our prayers as we would like. I shall never forget my grandmother teaching me this truth. She was a cripple, with one leg shorter than the other. As she got older she had more and more pain and in my opinion had cause to grumble. She was no saint, she was as human as you and I, but she was a very godly person. I loved her very much and was delighted when she came to live with us. I was then in my teens and I used to pray earnestly that God would heal my granny. It didn't seem quite fair that after she had been a missionary and given her life to Him in service, that he should let her suffer so. In my naiveté and idealism I began to believe that one day she would wake up with equal lengthed legs, that all her pain would have gone and that then she would be able to be an even greater witness of the goodness of God.

One day my grandmother was going to her son's for a fortnight's holiday. I don't know whether she had had a very painful night or whether it was just the sight of her limping away, but I stopped her and told her about my prayers. I said, 'Granny, I really believe God is going to heal you so that you are completely better.'

I shall always remember the smile on her face and the gentle way in which she explained that she did not believe that any longer. Once she had prayed the same prayer, once she had hoped and believed that God would heal her, but not any more. She told me that she had accepted her short leg and that it didn't really matter all that much any more, because she knew that one day she would be with the Lord, and then she would be whole. She told me not to weep for her handicap, but to praise God for all the good things He had given her in life.

I never saw my grandmother again. She died whilst on holiday with my uncle. Little though she knew it, she left me with an important truth and a lovely memory.

We have only to turn to the story of Paul to know again the truth of this. Although we do not know what was wrong with Paul, we do know that it was severe enough for him to pray repeatedly that God would remove it from him, because he felt it was a hindrance to him. Yet God did not and Paul was given instead the grace to accept it and live with it.[27]

I can theorize and talk and think up persuasive arguments, but in the end of the day I am now one of the 'haves'. I am no longer infertile or childless so whatever I believe, I can never speak from experience. Here is one who can. Marilyn and her husband could not have children of their own and know they never will have (although they have adopted). This is what she said to me.

'When things first began to go wrong, I was really miserable and when my friends and family hinted that maybe God didn't want us ever to have children of our own, I rejected it wholeheartedly. Later after several years and endless disappointments, I realized that we had come to the end of the line, that as a couple we were never going to have children of our own. I was devastated. There was only one possible way out, medically speaking, and that was AID, but I wouldn't even consider it, because I loved Alec and wanted his child, not some other man's.'

It was at this point, when there was no acceptable way open to them, that Marilyn and Alec had to stop and take stock. They had to start asking and answering a few basic questions, Marilyn explained what this meant:

'I realized that I had married Alec because I loved him and that in the end of the day he was more important to me than children. I dreaded widowhood far more than childlessness. God used this situation to draw the two of us even closer to each other. I found that I wanted to build Alec up, instead of criticizing him and vice versa. Our marriage was really enriched by all that we had been through.'

'United we stand' is a motto we could all take to heart, whatever our state. One of the marriage vows reminds us that we each need a special relationship with our marriage partner, which will stand up to the buffeting we receive, regardless of how the storm hits us.

> 'It was ordained for the companionship, help and comfort, which husband and wife ought to have of each other.'

In childlessness there are only two choices, to let God pull you together or to let go of God and fall apart. All the couples who shared their stories with me, whether or not they remained childless, admitted that the most important thing to do was to work through the agonies until you can come out with a right relationship with God and with each other.

Marilyn told me how she had fought long and hard to come to terms with God's harsh ruling and to accept the knowledge that she would never have her own genetic children.

'It took me a long time to accept that God really didn't want us to have children of our own. I was very rebellious and I had to pray daily about this, until finally God gave me the strength to accept it. When this happened I knew that it was a big step forward.'

What had Marilyn learnt through all this that she would like to pass on to others who have no hope of ever having a family?

'I think the most important thing you have to learn is to live with yourself and accept the situation as it is. You have to find out what God actually wants for you. You see, it is so easy to get caught up in the norm; marriage, a house, a mortgage, a car, a colour television, a video, a holiday abroad and a family. But is this actually God's norm, is this what He wants for you?'

So how do you go about coming to terms with yourself? From my own limited experience it is not easy to be objective, and positive. It is much easier to do a bit of shouting like Job did! How did Marilyn go about it?

'First, I had to get close to Him on a daily basis. I had to build a deeper relationship with Him and that means prayer and Bible study. Secondly, I had to accept my limitations, that is, the ones that He had given me. In other words, I had to accept that He had chosen to deny me children of my own and having done so to see what was possible within these limitations.'

'As a woman it is far more difficult to accept infertility, but I just had to come to terms with it and to realize that the Lord had something else in mind for me. I had to know in reality, with my heart as well as my head, that the Lord really does know what is best for me. Sometimes He seems to push us to our absolute limits, so that we are thrown back on Him and have to become utterly dependent on Him. It is only then that we let go in our own strength and so it is His strength which carries us through. It is only at this point that He can open our eyes to the opportunities and possibilities available to us.'

It is surely only when we are willing to surrender everything to God and to go on surrendering that He is able to bring peace and the ability to look forward and adapt to the childless lifestyle, not grudgingly, but graciously accepting God's purpose for our lives (albeit a different one from our dreams).

Recently a woman broke down when talking to me and cried, 'I will not give up. I cannot accept that God won't let me have a baby. It is my greatest desire.' She is still kicking against God and I grieve for what she is going through and will continue to go through until she can surrender to God's hand on the rein.

In Isaiah we read of a promise given to eunuchs, who have voluntarily given up their right to children, even as nuns and monks do today. I believe that when we surrender to God then we can take the same promise to ourselves,

> 'And let not any eunuch complain, 'I am only a dry tree'. For this is what the Lord says:
> 'To the eunuchs who keep my sabbaths, who choose what pleases me and hold fast to my covenant—to them I will give within my temple and its walls a memorial and a name better than sons and daughters; I will give them an everlasting name that will not be cut off.' Isaiah 56. 4b-5 (NIV)

This promise of an everlasting name should be a great

encouragement. Many people feel that by not giving birth, they have no stake in the future. They see only the pointlessness of a marriage without children, the loneliness of old age and the sadness of being the end of their particular line. I remember when we thought that we would never have children we were very aware that Ian was the only male member of our line of Cookes and that if we didn't pass on the name it would end a section of personal history. 'Genetic death' as it has been called can be a very soul-destroying thing for many people. However, as Christians we have a great hope for an everlasting future. Paul encourages us to look ahead with confidence,

> 'What is more I consider everything a loss compared to the surpassing greatness of knowing Christ Jesus my Lord, for whose sake I have lost all things . . . I want to know Christ and the power of his resurrection and the fellowship of sharing in his sufferings, becoming like him in his death, and so, somehow, to attain to the resurrection from the dead.' Philippians 3. 8, 10 (NIV)

Once you have accepted the finality of the situation, you are in a position to firmly close the door and open another one. After all you have been through you will have changed. You cannot be the same person you were when you got married. Inevitably you will be more mature, having survived the test. Now it is time to open another door and find out what God has in store for your life.

Once Marilyn had come to this point of acceptance, she was able to look ahead and start planning.

'I suppose you could say it is a bit like redundancy for a man. It can be a shattering experience to suddenly be without a job and it can be equally shattering to realize that you will never fulfil your original aim of having a child. Suddenly you have to apply your knowledge in quite a different framework. I found it was really exciting, because I realized that as a Christian the world really was my oyster! As a Christian, you are open to anything, but if you look only at what appears to be the norm it is a very narrow field. From society's viewpoint you are severely restricted but from God's viewpoint you have the whole world, literally, at your fingertips.'

'You have to lay yourself open to Him and what He has in store. It's awfully difficult to do. I know how hard it is, especially because of the pressures all around us to conform. We were desperate to be like our friends, but being a Christian isn't an insurance policy. It is a relationship with God the Father, the Son and the Holy Spirit. He chose not to heal us, either directly through the medical profession or miraculously. It is His will that we cannot have our own children and He has taught us so much through it.

'For example, I had always had everything I wanted, now I was denied the baby I longed for. I had always succeeded in everything, now I had tasted failure. Alec and I really grew up through this experience. Now I don't even want God to heal us, because I am sincerely grateful for the enriching of our lives and this is now more important to me.'

'The next step was to be positive about the future. What was I going to do, to fulfil my need and my desire for children? I thought seriously about helping in a home or playgroup with handicapped children. I wondered whether I should re-train, so that I could get a permanent job working with children, but meanwhile I took a temporary job with a Christian firm. As time went on we decided to try for adoption, before I went ahead with re-training.'

We are individuals. God has made us all different and consequently He has different plans for each one of us. Some people find fulfilment in their career. This is often the case for the man, who started life knowing that he would work until retirement. The daily toil takes the best part of the day, so it shouldn't be the 'daily grind'. If work isn't progressing as you expected, if you are unhappy or frustrated in it, then perhaps this is the time to look for something more fulfilling.

However, there is a danger in allowing the finality of childlessness or bereavement to encourage one to make the wrong decision. It is better to wait until you have come through the initial shock and can take a calmer, objective view and then make the right decision about changing jobs.

I know one man who changes his job every time a crisis hits his life, then wakes up in the aftermath to discover that he is no better off than before, having lost the stability and security of his familiar job. As in retirement people often rush into moving to a seaside resort or in early widowhood move in with their family, so in childlessness there is a danger in leaving secure and familiar places and situations because of temporary disillusionment.

It is much harder for the wife who expected to give up work to have a family and now finds that she has no 'excuse'. However, so many women choose to return to work soon after pregnancy, whilst others choose to delay having a family so that they can develop a career, that a woman should not feel too isolated or that she sticks out like a sore thumb. In fact, it is easier to be childless at work than at home, because so often the home situation leaves you surrounded by young families and the only mid-week openings are at mother and toddler groups and so on. It can be very lonely at home without children.

Whether full-time or part-time, the job you choose should be fulfilling and absorbing, offering good opportunities for your own personal scope. As you adjust to your unwanted freedom there may be other ways that you can use your time. Some people find extremely satisfying roles at church. It doesn't have to be with children or young people. You don't have to prove anything to anybody, so choose to do something that you will enjoy. One young couple in a local church have decided to use their lovely peaceful home. There can be a special blessing in a home that is not overrun by shouting children and scattered toys. This couple entertain somebody every single Sunday, two or three evenings a week and frequently have lonely students to stay. They have a real gift in making overseas people feel 'at home' in our country.

It may be that you have a desire to 'mother' new

Christians, or single folk. You have a good opportunity to keep open house at all hours, which couples with young families do not. Due to sleepless nights we try to be in bed by eleven o'clock, but many people are only just coming alive then and are ready to talk. If you can be a night owl you will be constantly in demand! God promises fulfilment:

> 'Sing, O barren woman, you who never bore a child; burst into song, shout for joy, you who were never in labour; because more are the children of the desolate woman than of her who has a husband,'
> says the Lord.
> Enlarge the place of your tent, stretch your curtains wide, do not hold back;
> lengthen your cords, strengthen your stakes.
> For you will spread out to the right and to the left;
> your descendants will dispossess nations and settle in their desolate cities.
> Do not be afraid, you will not suffer shame.
> Do not fear disgrace; you will not be humiliated.'
> Isaiah 54. 1-4a (NIV)

Despite the fact that Alec and Marilyn were pushed to the limits, she can now say,

'I have found that God can fill your whole life, if you have no children. He has given us back far more than He ever took from us.'

Accepting that you will never bear your own genetic child is one of the hardest things to do. God gave Alec and Marilyn the strength to endure and finally to accept His verdict. Sometimes the suffering seems hard and unfair, but Marilyn told me that she felt both privileged and cherished, in the proving of her faith;

> 'These (trials) have come so that your faith—of greater worth than gold, which perishes even though refined by fire—may be proved genuine and may result in praise, glory and honour when Jesus Christ is revealed.' 1 Peter 1. 7 (NIV)

We read in Scripture that God will never try us beyond our capabilities,

> 'So far you have faced no trial beyond what man can bear. God keeps faith, and He will not allow you to be tested above your powers, but when the test comes He will at the same time provide a way out, but enabling you to sustain it.'
>
> 1 1 Corinthians 10. 13 (NEB)

Marilyn radiated the joy of the Lord as she shared her experience with me. It was a real blessing to see how the Lord had healed her emotionally and spiritually and to see His hand in her life. She is a happy and contented woman, fulfilled in the mothering of her adopted children and in her witnessing for the Lord.

In retrospect most of us can rejoice in what the Lord has taught us through our experiences. Like Marilyn I had never really suffered failure and it was good for me to have to wait. I had never really had to stretch the elastic of my faith to see how far it would go, nor had I even had to question the God of love that I believed in.

I know now, through experience what Paul means when he says that testing brings maturity of character.

> '... we also rejoice in our sufferings, because we know that suffering produces perseverance; perseverance, character; and character, hope. And hope does not disappoint us because God has poured out His love into our hearts by the Holy Spirit whom He has given us.' (Romans 5. 3-5 NIV)

There comes a point for all of us, when God has allowed us to hit the depths of despair, when our pride is in the dust and we have no resources of our own left. Then we have two choices to give God the go-by or to acknowledge that we are empty, a mere nothing and that He is everything. When we admit that He is sovereign, the mighty and all-powerful ruler of the Universe, the Creator of our lives, who has a minute plan for each one of us, and our loving Father, then and only then, can He fill us and heal us, revive us and guide us, strengthen and renew us. But beware! We make no bargains with God, no sale or return of our allegiance. This is no barter or purchase that carries with it a guarantee that we will get what we want.

It must be unequivocal surrender to God, knowing that He has the right still to withold from you the baby you want. He will heal you spiritually and emotionally if you will let Him, but He may not heal you physically. Your only guarantee when you surrender completely to Him, is that He is faithful and loving and that whatever He plans for you, it is the best. As Marilyn said, 'God can fill your life.'

Practical hints on accepting total infertility

1 Recognize the end of the line. If there is a medical reason for it then this is easier to do. However, if no reason has been found for your infertility, then it is important for you and your husband to decide on an end. Otherwise the tensions created by living in a permanent state of hoping are liable to threaten all your other relationships.
2 Tell someone you respect and trust and ask them to pray for (and with) you during these early days of coming to terms with yourself.
3 Don't be afraid of your feelings; anger, rebellion against God or whatever. Admit to yourself, your husband and your confidant exactly what is going on inside. This is vital for true healing. (Try reading Job, especially chapters 3, 6, 7; 1 Samuel 1; Psalm 13; Psalm 22)
4 Get to know God intimately, by reading your Bible on a regular basis and talking to Him all the time.
5 Get to know yourself. If you're not besotted by children, don't feel you should be, there are no end of really fulfilling things to do with your life that do not involve children. If you do have a need and desire for children admit it and explore the ways that you might meet this need. Most important of all, don't be forced into a mould by anyone.
6 Fill your days. Is your job really fulfilling? If not,

consider a change. If you are not working look for something absorbing to do, preferably that helps others because that is so rewarding.

7 Move house. If you are on an estate overrun by young families and this is isolating you then be realistic about it and move. You don't have to stay put just to prove something.

8 Use your home. You may not wish to fill it with stray children, playing universal aunt, but there are still many openings; students, single people, other couples with infertility problems, OAPs who long to be part of a vibrant home again and so on.

9 Enjoy your freedom, even though you didn't choose it. Be positive. You will have more ready cash as well as more flexibility. You don't have to take holidays in school times so you could maybe afford to go abroad off-peak. Do something you couldn't do if you had children.

10 Expand your hobbies. Take up an evening class, or two! If you feel you can't get involved enough, try some voluntary work. There's a lot of help needed that can be done at 'hobby' level.

11 Use your experience if you can. Not everyone is cut out to be a counsellor, but everyone can listen and you can understand because you have been through a severe time of testing and have won through. Be ready if the opportunity arises.

12 On the days when the pain wells up again, don't be ashamed or feel that in some way you have failed. Allow yourself time to grieve again so that you can release yourself.

13 By now you should have some idea of what God has in mind for you. Get to it. Put your whole being into doing His will and remember that this is His best for you, never second best. Total healing will come as you lose yourself in Him.

Glossary of Terms

Abortion

Technically the expulsion of a foetus during the first 12 weeks of pregnancy, whether spontaneous or induced. Common usage is for the delivery of a non-viable foetus in the first 28 weeks of pregnancy.

Artificial Insemination

The injection of semen into the uterus using artificial means. The semen specimen is drawn into a syringe, which is attached to a straw-sized metal cannula, and inserted in the vagina, where it is flushed over the cervix several times.

Artificial Insemination Donor (AID)

Insemination with sperm provided by a donor.

Artificial Insemination Homologous (AIH)

Insemination with the husband's sperm.

Basal Body Temperature (BBT)

Temperature taken first thing in the morning before getting out of bed. If taken regularly at the same time it should be roughly the same each day. Thus the increase due to ovulation will be readily noticeable.

Bromocriptine

A drug that acts directly on the pituitary surpassing the production of prolactin and increasing the levels of FSH. It induces ovulation and menstruation and may increase sperm formation.

Cervix

Neck of the uterus.

Clomiphene Citrate or Clomid

A fertility pill, which stimulates ovulation. Clomid stimulates the hypothalamus to instruct the pituitary to produce FSH, which in turn triggers the development and release of an egg. It is only successful in women who have adequate levels of oestrogen, can manufacture FSH and have healthy ovaries.

Dilatation and Curettage (D&C)

A small operation in which the cervical canal is dilated and the uterine cavity is scraped with a curette, which is a small spoon-shaped instrument.

Embryo
The fertilized egg from the moment of fertilization until the twelfth week.

Fallopian Tubes (also called oviducts)
Tubes connecting the ovaries to the uterus. Funnel shaped for the transport of eggs and the site of fertilization.

Fertilization
The union of the egg and the sperm.

Follicle-stimulating Hormone (FSH)
A hormone produced by the pituitary gland in both men and women. In women it is cyclical to stimulate the maturation of the egg and its follicle. In men it stimulates sperm cell formation and maturation.

Galactosaemia
The deficiency of an enzyme required for the utilization of glucose in the body. It can be successfully treated by excluding lactose and galactose from the diet. Some mental and physical retardation may occur depending on the time of diagnosis and success of treatment.

Gene
The hereditary factors present in a definite position on a particular chromosome. Controls a particular inherited characteristic of an individual.

Genetic Incompatibility
The genes contributed by the male and female are unable to exist together and therefore tend to create a malformed human being.

Hormones
Chemical substances produced by the endocrine glands to regulate various body mechanisms.

Human Chorionic Gonadotropic Hormone (HCG)
Hormone produced by the placenta during pregnancy. It is used as the basis of pregnancy tests.

Infertility
Primary infertility is the inability to achieve a pregnancy after one year of unprotected, unlimited intercourse. Secondary infertility is the inability to carry a pregnancy to birth and is also the term applied to those women who have conceived before

and given birth to a child, but who are unable to conceive again.

It is estimated that approximately 15% of the adult population in the child-bearing group suffers from primary infertility. If you include those suffering from secondary infertility then there may be some three million affected couples in the UK.

In Vitro Fertilization (IVF)

The fertilization of an egg by sperm, in a test-tube. The egg is removed from the woman, fertilized in the test-tube and then returned to the womb for implantation.

Laparoscopy

Examination of the abdominal cavity with a laparoscope, which is like a telescope, inserted through a small incision into the abdominal cavity. Carbon dioxide gas is inserted via a needle inserted at the umbilicus, to blow out the organs for better visibility. A dye inserted through the cervix should be seen coming out of the fallopian tubes.

Luteinizing Hormone

Emitted by the pituitary gland in men and women. Cyclical in women to stimulate the formation of the corpeus luteum, which manufactures progesterone. In men it develops the cells of the testicles that produce the male hormone testosterone.

Miscarriage

Technically the expulsion of a foetus between the fourth and sixth month of pregnancy. Common usage is the spontaneous termination of a pregnancy before 28 weeks.

Oestrogen

Female hormone formed by the developing egg.

Oligospermia

Low sperm count—less than 20 million sperm per ml. (norm. 20-200 million)

Ovary

Reproductive organ of the female, which produces eggs.

Ovulation

The release of the egg from the ovary. Usually occurs

about the fourteenth day of the woman's menstrual cycle, in a normal 28 day cycle.

Pergonal
A fertility pill. The hormone FSH is extracted from the urine of post-menopausal women. It acts directly on the ovaries to cause ovulation and carries a high risk of multiple pregnancy.

Primolut
A natural progesterone, given by injection in the early weeks of pregnancy.

Progesterone
Female hormone secreted by the corpeus luteum. Important in the regulation of the menstrual cycle and during pregnancy. It is important in the formation of the lining of the uterus, which feeds the fertilized egg. Inadequate progesterone may cause early miscarriage.

Prolactin
A hormone, which if present in excess may cause failure of the menstrual cycle and may be indicative of a brain tumour. It may affect sperm formation if present in excessive quantities in the male.

Post Coital Test
Examination of the cervical mucus shortly after intercourse to discover whether cervical mucus and sperm are compatible.

Sperm Count
A test to determine the number and nature of sperm produced by the male. Can be subject to illness which may depress the sperm count. At least three checks should be done at different times.

Sperm Morphology
The shape of sperms. All normal men have 10% abnormal sperms. The requirement for fertility is 60% normal.

Sperm Motility
Ability of sperm to move. Thought to be the single most important aspect of sperm quality. It is thought that excellent motility will increase the chances of pregnancy even in a low count. Norm: 60-85% active, one hour after ejaculation.

Tomography

X-ray at different levels within the skull. Used for examination of the pituitary gland.

Uterus

The womb. A pear-shaped hollow organ situated at the top of the vagina in which the fertilized egg implants and the baby grows.

Varicocele

Varicose veins in the scrotal sac. Reduces the sperm count. Surgical removal improves the sperm count in about 75% of cases and the pregnancy rate by about 45%.

Venereal Disease

Infection transmitted primarily during intercourse.

References

1 Orders and Prayers for Church Worship (1960) p 184ff Baptist Union.
2 Stanway, Andrew (1980) '*Why Us?*' Granada Publishing Ltd.
3 The Free Church Federal Council and The British Council of Churches (1982) *Choices in Childlessness* (London).
4 Hall, Katherine (1983) '*Learning to Cope with Childlessness*' p 2 A.R. Mowbray and Co. Ltd.
5 Newsweek (December 6th 1982) No. 49 pp 34-41.
6 *Choices in Childlessness* p 29.
7 *Learning to Cope with Childlessness* p 6.
8 Luke 18. 1-6
9 *Why Us?* pp 135-137.
10 IBID p 125.
11 CHILD, Infertility Research, Education and Counselling. Charity.
12 NAC, National Association for the Childless and Childfree.
13 Donald, Ian *et al* (1984) '*Test Tube Babies—a christian view*' p iii. Unity Press, Becket Publications.
14 IBID p 28.
15 Jaeck, Gordon and Dorothea (1967), '*Take My Marriage*', p 89, Lakeland.
16 Eareckson, Joni (1976), '*Joni*', pp 138, 149, Pickering and Inglis.
17 Ten Boom, Corrie (1971), '*The Hiding Place*', pp 184-185, Hodder and Stoughton.
18 *Choices in Childlessness* p vii.
19 DHSS, Dame Mary Warnock (1984), Report of the Committee of Inquiry into Human Fertilization and Embryology. HMSO. ISBN 0 10 193140 9.
20 IBID pp 32-34.
21 IBID pp 37-38.
22 IBID pp 40-41.
23 Dobson, James C. (1981) '*Straight Talk To Men and Their Wives.*' Hodder and Stoughton.
24 Warnock Report pp 23-28.

25 IBID pp 24-25.
26 IBID p 19.
27 IBID pp 46-47.
28 Learning to Cope with Childlessness pp 9-10.
29 Mark 14. 36.
30 1 Samuel 1. 20. Samuel means 'asked of the Lord.'

Useful Addresses

CHILD
Farthings
Gaunts Rd
Pawlett
Nr Bridgewater
Somerset
Tel: 0278 683595

NATIONAL ASSOCIATION for the CHILDLESS
318, Summer Lane
Birmingham B19 3RL
Tel: 021-359 4887

BRITISH AGENCIES for ADOPTION and FOSTERING
11 Southwark Street
London SE1 1RQ
Tel: 01-407 8800

MISCARRIAGE ASSOCIATION
Dolphin Cottage
4, Ashfield Terrace
Thorpe
Nr Wakefield
W. Yorks WF12 9QH
(Please include *s.a.e.*)

NATIONAL CHILDBIRTH TRUST (Have produced a booklet on miscarriage)
5 Queensborough Terrace
London W2 3TB